T0064315

RACISM WITH SUBSTANCE INDUCED MOOD DISORDERS

Aneb Jah Rasta Sensas-Utcha Nefer I

Order this book online at www.trafford.com
or email orders@trafford.com

Most Trafford titles are also available at major online book retailers.

Print information available on the last page.

ISBN: 978-1-4907-6463-4 (sc)
ISBN: 978-1-4907-6462-7 (e)

Trafford rev. 08/25/2015

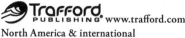 www.trafford.com
North America & international
toll-free: 1 888 232 4444 (USA & Canada)
fax: 812 355 4082

SUBSTANCE INDUCED MOOD DISORDERS INVOLVING RACE AND RACISM

Racism has polluted the soul of all living things of existence. This is from the story of the so-called deception within the Garden of Eden. You know who was in the garden. It was Ausar and Auset of Khamit. However, the European Japhite has denounced the Black man ever since that KJV Bible and prior to it being written. As Easter is a holiday for the Christian, it has its day which is different each year. Did Jesus die on different days each year? Was this originally Passover? Why is the day of Easter different every year! This is from the leader of the Nation of Islam. Although, I am not a member of the Nation of Islam, I must say, "I agree". This is wholly paganism.

Hosea 4:6 Therefore, the people perish due to the lack of knowledge. In many cases, this is a variety of instances of intentional forms of ignorance. Individuals have often played on ignorant as they have continued in their own arrogance and psychical schemes of the paganistic heathen. In this, they have become ill by their own schemes. Schemes of such as racisms and wholly forms of wickedness. Wickedness, by forms of vile and profane lusts. Lusts in being aware of their situation(s). However, in their situation(s) they exclude important knowledge of the true God. The true god is Ausar is within all men and women. This has been a hidden agenda by the manipulated and conditioned church and physician of the western civilization.

Surah 20:102 we shall gather the guilty, blue-eye on that day. This is in reference to the guilty being raised up blind in the Resurrection. In verse 124 mentions that 'we shall raise him or her up blind in the day of Resurrection. This individual does not receive spiritual blessings due to his or her own intent of misleading through internal wickedness, seduction, perversion and ill-prosperous motives of Set. Therefore, resurrection is the capturing of one's individual spirit and soul and becoming aware of the darkness that was once in his or her life. In this, recognition is potentialized by the understanding of his or her own divinity. The divinity that has been hindered by deliberate forms of cognitive sin. In cognitive sin, there are unawares that occur. These unawares are forms of intentional sin.

You see, this may seem contrary to the core. To the core of one's own destruction in sin. This is deliberate sin. In deliberate sin, there are various forms of discrimination. In discrimination, there are several factors that are manifested. Manifested by heathanistic methodologies of idolatry, paganism and racism. You see, this is biblical, religious and spiritual. In the biblical sense, there is hatred and deliberate forms of racism and discrimination that begins in the book of Genesis to Revelation. The bible denounces race relations with the African. However, it incorporates unity regarding other races and religious groups / sects. In this, this is an interdependent form of exclusion of the Black. As the biblical scholars and writers had intentionally excluded the so-called minority for centuries up to this very day. They, the Caucasian has sold out other races since the origin of communication efforts with mankind.

As mentioned in the NAMI – Peer to Peer guide, this tells us that this is something beyond genes that are involved in the development of mental illness. You see, mental illness is racial as well as religious, spiritual and political. Therefore, this is a pathogen of generational curses as well as pure forms of deliberate arrogance and ignorance regarding the lives of all people. Just look @ Cliven Bundy and the modern GOP. This has been a scheme of bigotry, fraud, hatred and racism since the inclusion of politics in the America's and throughout the entire world. In this, higher forms of hypocrisy are reconstructed.

This is, as the Bible wasn't written for the benefit of Black people, meaning the Africans. In this, as Ezekiel prophesized regarding the Valley of The Dry Bones so shall the lost be reconciled with the true living God. You see, Japheth and Shem were nations of the Arab and Caucasian. In this, we find colonialism, hatred, racism and slavery. This was legal as nations were divided in order of maintaining divisions of races by legalizing slavery and permitting racism. Also, in the book (4 Centuries of Black Life, African American History) it was written that Blacks were Christianized and the Bible was a dangerous books. Indeed, that book was written by homosexuals. They were Langston Hughes and Milton Metzler.

Back to my point! You see, Africans were feared. Therefore, their instruments were forbidden. Mainly, their drums. As planters feared that by reading the Bible, Africans would cause riots and divisions amongst the house-nigga and the field nigga. In this, Shem is the Father of the Arabs. This is true, as the Arabs resided along the Asian Minor. They intermingled with the sons of Japheth along the Northern parts of Africa and the Southern parts of Europe. This is where the Greeks and Assyrians united and conquered African nations. You see, modern Russia is at odds with its own people. As Vladimir Putin had formed allies with enemies of Barak Obama and The United States of America. This is, in order to create nuclear weapons.

This is written in Ezekiel chapters 37 through 39. Of course, there are racial connotations to this scenario. The scenario is that there will always be forms of racial hatred and bigotry as long as Bibles are written and read by false preachers and so-called educators of world history. This is a theory of a much greater conspiracy against God. These are crimes against God! These are acts of grandeur and delusion. In this, there has been no solution for immigration rights nor human rights. How can there be human rights if there is no civility. There will never be peace in this Setianistic world of ideological slavery and bigotry. This is all about economics and the wealth of the ignorant and arrogant European and Arab.

You see, Japheth's Britons and Celtics have traced their royal houses from Japheth. If that is the case, the earliest bibles were written by explorers of colonialism, cannibalism and hypocrisy. This is a major travesty that will continue to enslave and plague current and future generations. This has led to terrorism and the Al Qaeda in the entire continent of modern Africa as well as European colonies and countries. You see, Ukraine, Russia and the Nigeria governments are similar and yet are in contrast towards each other. In this, this is a game of political football. This has led to slayings, racism within race and kidnappings amongst their people. This is an emotional form of genocide. Genocide as written in Ezekiel chapters 34 – 38 has been prophesied and fulfilled. However, The Valley of The Dry Bones must be resurrected by bringing out God's greatness. God's greatness is an interdependence of intelligence. This has nothing to do with idol worship as the Bible states. You see, in Deuteronomy 18 is states that one cannot call out omens and or worship the dead. Also, read Galatians 4:10. This specifically mentions that special days and times aren't to be worshipped.

What then is Black history month or the Westernized civilized holidays! This also includes a presidential holiday and or a special day for a dead individual who was and is recognized as famous. For example Michael Jackson or Abraham Lincoln. You see, this is remembrance. In remembering, you are focusing on the qualities and greatness of an individual(s).

In the African culture and religious practice, heritage and culture are recognized by the accomplishments of its people. This is a people of greatness in history that have not been recognized by the modern Caucasian, Arab and House-nigga African. You see, in this, there have been lynching and genocide of the mind and entire being on earth. Worship is nothing but calling out a special noun in order to receive a timely response. However, in unction there is a special capacity and knowledge that is required of an individual. This individual is then considered a Shechem, Priest, King or a Queen Mother within the African culture and religious practice.

Therefore, in awakening the Valley of The Dry bones in the Ausarian religion, Auset, the wife of Ausar, found the dismembered fourteen pieces of Ausar. You see, Set, who is Ausar's brother envied him and sliced him into fourteen pieces and murdered him. There is more to the entire story.

Therefore, through spiritual ritual a resurrection occurs. The body is equal to that of the universe. Equal to the molecular and periodic elemental forces of the universe. In this, we find our connection to God! For, we are in the image and likeness of God. This is not what the Bible or Quran teaches us. However, the two books slightly mentions the fact that we are gods. That we are in the image and likeness of God. God is monotheistic. However, the books reveal that we are not. Therefore, you cannot have your cake and eat it. This is a shameful and legal form of organized slavery, hatred and racism within race. You see, we are divided on all forms of civilization. Therefore, God's love is universal love. However, hatred and economical forms of greed has enslaved the mind of the arrogant and ignorant by ostracism and torture. Jude 1:10 these people slander things that they do not understand. By this, there is misconceptions of their misunderstandings. Therefore, we realize that negations and forms of discrimination is their only way of life. In their lives they are inconsistent with regards to their own religion. Yet their religion is of dogmatic forms of delusions and grandeur. In this, they fail to recognize their god. Their god is an image of idolatry and fallacy.

It's fiction is of false hope and make-believing forms of faith. They pray for forgiveness, yet their behaviors aren't improved mechanisms of their weakened methods of conditionings. Their conditions are impulses of darkness. They have no love within them. They have no knowledge of their lives. They too are fanatical in their mental and spiritual slavery due to their self-indulging unawares of reality. They are heathens of their own circumstances. Their circumstances are eternities of the hells of the dry bones.

In this, racisms occur before our very eyes. Before our very eyes. We haven't held the notion of freedom due to our ignorance of world affairs. Of spiritual affairs as well as mental affairs. We are enslaved due to our close-mindedness. We have been suicidal daily. This is due to the lack of devotion, trust, love and understanding of humanity. Humanity is a gift from heaven to God. This is wisdom that I speak. This is not of arrogance combined with insanity. In arrogance and insanity we have a lost and a dying civilization. A civilization that allows the Devil to manipulate the lower parts of our being. The lower parts of our being deals with the sahu man and spirit. In this, we are disharmonized by subliminal messages that are known as psychological and spiritual triggers. So cut the crap. You European and Arabs are aware of this. This is an uncaring, cruel and selfish world.

From Satan, to the caveman unto modern civilization, we have been in denial. Denial of the fact that anything mixed with the African race is of the Afrocentric race. You see, we've lost our understanding of God's divinity. The divinity of God is within every living creature. Every living creature has a purpose within its origin and habitat. Truly, alcoholism and other drug related incidents, accidents and flaws have been major episodes of unethical schemes of the human race. In the Quran – Surah 4:43 it says - go not near prayer when you are intoxicated till you know what to say. Therefore, this leads to disaster of the human race. This which is the cause and stem of lust, perversion and greed. In this, there is a varied form of disaster and disorder. Disorder, by the means of disaster. Disaster leads to mood, emotional, cognitive and dysfunctions of anxiety.

You see! You are probably asking yourself the following question; "what does this have to do with racism"? Well, as The DSM mentions – racism is a mental illness. In fact, it really is a mental disorder. Children at a young age are taught this in cultures and educational systems throughout the world. All cultures are negligent due to their ignorance regarding history, current events and religious cultures. You see, this leads to major forms of depression and hatreds. We have been fooled to believe that the Caucasian has created all things. It was them, along with the Jew, Arab and House-nigga that were all drunkards, child molesters, criminals and murderers. This currently exist. This is universal slavery.

Mental slavery has been a betrayal within every sense of the word! Therefore, by an individual being strong in the physical sense doesn't make one totally whole. Wholeness brings a great deal of balance within the body, mind and spirit. A holistic individual is one who is in acceptance of The Tree of Life and The Tree of Knowledge Meditation System. To understand this, it takes a great deal of patience, dedication, love, trust and will. Effort is the key to longevity. In this, knowing that you are in the essence of God is essential in one's spiritual growth and development!

In knowing the above, the individual has the power to withstand the physical and spiritual boundaries that has been place before him/her. In this, the individual is capable of carrying out and maintaining self-control when faced with conditions of the external. Indeed, one is able to recognize directly what he or she is being faced with. The behaviors that need to be reshaped with spiritual healing. You see, there are various kinds of moods as well as depression. However, there is rarely a topic of discussion as it pertains to racism – substance induced mood disorders.

Well, African psychology verses European psychology differs a great deal. In addition, the African civilization has been faced with hatred, racism, slavery and a treacherous form of treatment at the hands of the European. This is what the DSM has failed to include in its manuals. Its manual doesn't discuss the topic of racism being a mental disorder. However, it is. On page 103 of DSM-5, it discusses Culture-Related Diagnostic Issues that are to be considered. However, in many cases they are often misinterpreted by the psychologist and or psychiatrist. In this, there are individuals who are unaware of cultural differences due to intentional forms of ignorance, discrimination and racism. Therefore, the clinician and patient has lost an opportunity of positive sharing. This often leads to the patient becoming induced with a variety of forms of substance abuse.

It says that cultural and socioeconomic factors must be considered when neither, the clinician and the patient do not share the same and cultural economic background. In this, individuals are often misdiagnosed. Although the individual may have a mental disability; However, to what extreme! Religious content must be understood.

What I am saying is "psychiatry is taught of the Maslow / Freudian view! Non-holistic approaches have enslaved and improperly shaped the lives of individuals who are living in poverty who have a mental illness(s).

Antipsychotic, antidepressants and mood enhancing medications are provided to improve the individual's being, mental and emotional state. However, in many cases, individuals are often rebellious towards their psychiatrists. In this, I am saying that Individuals turn to illicit drugs and other forms of substance in order to feel short term forms of relief. In addition; after being brainwashed during the embedding of false religious doctrines- / individuals have then turned to drug and substance abuse. In this, individuals are often introduced to the following; pornography, adultery and fornication. This is their way of escaping the so-called miseries of the world. Some individual often attempt to commit crimes, murder and suicide.

Suicide can occur within the spirit as well as in a physical sense. Indeed, in 1 Samuel 31; Apostle Paul / Saul asked to be murdered after attempting suicide. He too, in 1 Samuel 28 sought after a medium @ Endor. This is of which previously and later denied the use of such practice towards his followers. This occurred while Saul attempted to invoke the powers of Samuel. As well as during slavery and the conquest of Khamit and Canaan. Whereas; captains of all slave ships were induced with disease, tobacco, marijuana, opium and alcohol during their travels throughout the world. Canaan is modern Syria and Iraq. This too was known as Nineveh of the Old Testament during the pre-Israeli reign.

Therefore, hypocrisy is too a mental illness. This a contagious disease. Lying is a contagious disease of narcissism. The two are coincides towards each other. They are violations of Gods divine law. Yet, Paul says that we are redeemed from the curse of the law on several instances in the Holy Bible including Galatians 3:13. You read for yourselves the truth of the matter. You cannot have your cake and eat it. Choose whom you shall as written in Joshua. However, Joshua too, devised along with the Israelis succeeded in their plans to invade and slowly conquer Canaan. This was done by brainwashing, murdering, raping and enslaving its' youth and women.

INTOXICATION

You see, it can take seconds, minutes, hours and or days to trigger one's cognitive and emotional state of being. In this, the neurotransmitters and receptors of the brain receives energy from each other. This is stimuli. Stimuli causes an individual to respond to various forms of activity. This is called Nekhebet and Uatchet of the Khamitic Religious tradition. In this, these are unseen forces that can eventually harm and dismantle one's entire being, spirit and soul. This may seem to be contrary according to the books of Galatians and Colossians. You see, the two books discuss the use religious philosophies that are induced with elemental powers and spiritual forces by the traditions of men. However, this is contrary within its' own sense as written in the Bible. Indeed, tradition means ancestry. Therefore, throughout the African culture and civilization there has a history of ancestry worship. Numbers 23:9 as slavery has postponed the African from having a greater awareness and knowledge of God.

Yeah, indeed, and truly, Paul discusses his ancestry and culture throughout the New Testament. As an example, in Acts 28:17 Paul mentions that he's done nothing against his own people or ancestry. That's a lie: As King Saul, I he was a murderer, drunkard, who persecuted and robbed the church. The majority of the New Testament was written by Paul. Therefore, who are you worshipping.

Back to my point! Intoxication is a violation of the divine law of God. It causes various disorders. In this, there are several factors. First of all, one's emotional state is often deterred. Head trauma is often developed. Also, individuals will have impaired speech. Yes, this is a very serious impairment. Oxygen levels of the brain become extremely dysfunctional. Therefore, there are instances of both auditory and visual hallucinations. This leads to perversions, fornication, adultery and idolatry. In addition, unseen forces, such as hidden enemies will lay wait to devour your being with strong intentions of harm that lays within the demonic realm. Individuals often lurk in their passion to dissolve your character, spirit and being whenever you are intoxicated.

You see, intoxication leads to sedated thought processes. Here is what I am getting at. Intimacy shouldn't occur when an individual is intoxicated whether it is a result of alcohol or another form of drug. Intimacy should occur with the mutual understanding of trust. However, in modernity – there is a form of idolatry and ideation. This is of a passion that is grandeur. Passion can be of grandeur. However, it must be of love. In addition, this often leads to emotional distress and depression mood disorders. Mood disorders are then of the substance induced factor. Therefore, intoxication leads to children who are innately induced with brain diseases and mental disorders.

In many cases, Idiosyncratic Disorder is the use of a small amount of alcohol by an individual. This causes the individual to become easily impaired. According to the DSM III, this particular individual has amnesia and usually becomes belligerent and assaultive. In this, trauma and encephalitis occurs. This individual also becomes epileptic, cancerous and anemic with sickle cell. Note: the individual also has signs of Alzheimer's, Parkinson, Neuroleptic Induced Disorder and or Dementia.

You see, the spirit is also a powerful spirit. In the Khamitic religion, individuals violate the laws of Sekert, Herukhuti and Maat by the overindulgence of alcohol and other recreational drugs and medication. As previously mentioned, in the realm of Nekhebet and Uatchet, there are elemental forces that fall in the line of unseen enemies. Enemies of the spiritual realm are on the prowl to devour you by seducing the lower portion of your spirit that within the Tree of Life and the Tree of Knowledge Meditation System. They know your strengths and weaknesses according to astrological charts. However, astrology does not control one's destiny. You – God does.

Everyone is in the likeness and image of God. Therefore, it is the responsibility of every individual to seek his or her own salvation with the understanding that he or she is in the image and likeness of God. However, sin entered the world in Genesis – yet was redeemed in the book of Revelation. I beg to differ. You the European – Japath and Arab Shem poisoned the African people after enslaving them and trading them for gin, rum and other offensive intoxicants.

Therefore, alcoholism leads to sexual inappropriateness and or aggression, mood swings, agitation, speech impairment, impaired judgment and stupor / comatose. You see, in this, there are mechanisms of aggression which leads to MDD, bipolar, schizophrenia and other behavioral dysfunctions in prenatal stages of development. Such as infant death syndrome. Children tend to suffer severely due to them being the offspring. Indeed, this is genetic. In genetics, we find that there are factors that have proven the biblical scholars to be correct. As they have written that these are generational curses. Although, the culture of biblical studies weren't written for the benefit of all people. That is to say The African, Asian and Latino. As you can see! If you have studied any form of history, all of them are of the African heritage.

What are generational curses? Generational curses are due to individuals and certain cultures lacking the true knowledge of its own culture. This can be of its religious, culture, society and ancestry. In most cases, individuals have no understanding of his or her own destiny. This leads to psychiatric betrayal, mental slavery, self-denial as well as self-hatred. In addition, individuals then turn to alcoholism and drug abuse. This often leads to racially offensive remarks. This occurs throughout an individuals' social and personal life.

Back to my point with regards to generational curses as they relate to alcoholism. Alcoholism can be and is genetically linked. In this, various birth defects occur. Sudden Infant Death Syndrome as well as ADHD occurs within the child. The child might have to see a speech pathologist. The child might have cerebral palsy. The child might even have chronic brain dysfunction, schizophrenia, various forms of bipolar along with developmental disabilities.

History is something that cannot be forgotten. It must be taught at all times. The Asian and African has a rich ancestry. In this, we must recognize the facts and fallacies behind the education of the prenatal – adolescent and adult. Throughout alcoholism, there are triggers. This occurs throughout any form of addiction. However, this addiction leads to Major Depressive Disorders. This is where individuals will do anything to feed their alcoholic addiction. They'll lie, cheat and steal to maintain ease their emotional state. What I am saying is; that they'll become extremely belligerent and extremely emotional when encountering an episode.

Denial is their escape. They become scapegoats by blaming others for their wrongdoings. They are then extremely emotional and externally opposed to treatment. Their spirit becomes somber. Their depression worsens. While on the other hand, their sex drive is enhanced. They have a variety of sexual partners. Within this, STD's enter their bloodstream. Their disability deepens. Their denial becomes extreme. As crazy and weird as this seems, this is a form of truth of which I am writing. DSM 3 page 128 mentions that more than one-half of all murderers and their victims are believed to have been intoxicated at the time of the act. Also ¼ of suicides occur while the person is drinking alcohol.

Note, loquacity and increased sociability occurs along with irritability and an impaired judgment due to alcohol intoxication. Alcoholism can suppress immune mechanisms and cause other infections such as TB and Diabetes. There are predisposing factors such as malnutrition and chronic fatigue syndrome. In this, alcohol hallucinations develop during stages of withdrawal. Indeed, sweating, hyperactivity, seizures and irregular tremors occur within hands, tongue and eyelids.

Malaise due to alcohol withdrawal leads to vomiting, headaches and nausea. In this, individuals tend to have fevers and or hot flashes. This is a form of myalgia. You see, there are several factors in this. In addition, individuals have extreme urges of addiction due to extreme and subtle changes in their anatomy. Their anatomy becomes extremely discomforted by instant and constant urges of alcohol and other harmful substances. Harmful substances can be of the prescribed medicinal type / street drugs. In this, people become induced with nicotine, marijuana, crack - / cocaine and the abuse of painkillers. This also includes heroin addiction in teens and young adults. This is most common in suburban areas verses the inner city.

This leads to teen pregnancy and sudden infant death syndrome as a result of jaundice. Jaundice is when both eyes and skin color becomes yellow. In this, major episodes of mania, delusion, chronic brain dysfunction, cerebral palsy, MS and or other dysfunctions arise within the cerebral cortex of the unborn child.

There are diseases that occur such as hepatitis, sickle cell anemia, HPV, HIV, AIDS, TB and various cancers. This also includes liver cancer, lung cancer, Tongue Cancer, Throat Cancer, Mouth Cancer, colorectal cancer, pancreatic cancer and others. Post Nasal Drip Disorder is another factor along with mesothelioma. The two are induced by the inhalation of chemicals, acids and dust from second hand marijuana and cigarette smoke. They are also caused by saran - and gases in household and cleaning supplies. Those diseases are also caused by individuals not drinking enough water. These two are disorders that are caused by the over usage of dairy products or lack of protein and calcium thereof.

In many cases, too many medications can cause those harmful symptoms of discomfort. This can include one or all of the following; diabetes, heart disease and or anxiety. The following are consequences of alcoholism and drug abuse. This relates to ancestral disorders. In ancestral disorders there are pathogens through genes and disorders of chromosomes. You see, COPD is chronic obstructive pulmonary disease. In this, this too is a form of asthma and bronchitis. This is of which in individual's bronchial tubes have lost oxygen. Loss of oxygen can eventually lead to brain tumors, alzhiemers, dementia and or parkinson's disease. Memory loss is also the early stages of the previous sentence.

By the individual enhancing the mantras Geb and Auset , he or she will become capable of managing his or her chi, life-force. Through meditation and exercise, the individual will eventually become capable of subduing many forms of disease and bodily dysfunction. However, westernization has been the central theme of medical manslaughter and murder of the African community. In this, physicians first gained their knowledge from ancient Kemet and Canaan. However, they have failed to give credit where credit is due. Therefore, the cancer of humankind has left the poor and indignant with confusion, self-hatred, denial and isolation. See Deuteronomy 28:28 where it says that you'll be left in blindness and confusion.

Ask your person the following; if I am in the image of God, will I allow those things to happen to me knowing that I am in the likeness of God. Therefore, the biblical scholars got this one incorrect when they wrote the bible. This is a carcinogen of darkness that has left our ancestors in an artery of disparity. This artery of disparity is bipolar mania. In bipolar mania, alcoholism at oftentimes leads to urinary tract infections, gall bladder infections along with kidney and liver diseases.

This is from the overexcitement of neurons and nerves of the PNS and CNS. Through heredity, there are symptoms of immunological diseases. These diseases include IBD, HIV and AIDS. Therefore, anxieties occur that causes strokes and heart attacks. Stress occurs due to poor nutrition, lack of proper diet and lack of spiritual development. Whenever an individual lacks spiritual development, he or she lacks the understanding of the health laws that are guided by and through meditation.

Therefore, alcohol abuse is an escape and defense mechanism that is used by those who are looking for a self-fulfilling prophecy that usually goes unfulfilled. That is, the broken hearted. This has specifically devised for the nonwestern individual to fail. In failing, the true man, woman and child of God suffers wrongfully. You see, no one is to suffer. Especially if the individual has become aware the he or she is a god and in the likeness of God. Therefore, no one person is going to die for the sake of all through beatings and acts of torture of the flesh. The world has been bewitched by the hands of the Setien. The Setien has lied before the bible was written and will continue to deceive.

The prostrate of darkness has left billions of our ancestors in their deathbed at the hands of the heathenistic slaver. Maat is the catalyst for divine development of judgment. In her judgment, she disallows individuals to overindulge in immoral acts. The majority of the acts of immorality deals with perverse behaviors. In perverse behaviors there is alcoholism and drug abuse. This leads to bladder diseases and sexual prowess.

This is also a form of autoimmune hepatitis. Hepatic Granulomas can be tumors that are within the liver, Syphilis, Chronic Fatigue Syndrome and or the genealogical rabbit / animal disease – Francisella Tubarenis. In the listed diseases and disorders, we find that feces and blood pathogens are often linked to sexually transmitted diseases. Truly, there are serious consequences resulting from alcoholism, poor hygiene and individuals living in an unclean living environment.

FETAL ALCOHOL SYNDROME (FAS)

(FAS) is abnormalities associated with the mother's using alcohol during pregnancy; defects range from mild to severe, including growth retardation, brain damage, mental retardation, hyperactivity, facial anomalies and heart failure. Infants are often born with viral infections such as aids, herpes and or syphilis. This disorder is also called alcohol embryopathy. this, Fetal Alcohol Syndrome also causes physical deformities. In addition, in animal toxicology in rabbits teratology studies, temperatures drop in them when given alcohol / - adrenalin. There is shock within the caritoid vein and artery. This often includes dysfunctions within the jugular vein.

In addition, psychoactive drugs overlap with other drugs as it relates to combination therapy. In combination therapy, the ANS, PNS and CNS are often damaged and or destroyed. Therefore, it is encouraged that there is to be no alcohol or other drug use to occur during pregnancy. However, in many cases doctors often prescribe medications to nursing mothers without informing them of the consequences of drug intake. This often leads to a child being born with (ARND) Alcohol Related Neurodevelopmental Disorders and he or she is often diagnosed with attachment disorders, conduct and behavioral disorders.

In this, there are complications with the antidepressant medication Depakote, Lithium as well as Ritalin. Depakote is a mood stabilizer that causes various birth defects and chromosomal dysfunctions. It can be taken as a form of birth control pill. In addition, Depakote is human growth hormone that interferes with an individual's normal sleep pattern. Hormone dysfunction is a vital discomfort to patients while taking Depakote. This stearate causes tremors and males to have female breast.

Therefore, individuals who have been diagnosed as alcoholics are often in denial. However, they'll do anything for a drink. They're like infants who are crying to be fed with a bottle or breast. In addition, various forms of childhood cancerous viruses occur along with along with the development of juvenile diabetes. You see, along with embryopathy there is a pattern of diseases such as HPV, HIV and Aids. In this, there are other pathogenic diseases and disorders such as bone marrow diseases chronic brain disorders.

Leukemia occurs due to tumors of the brain as it relates to Bone Mineral Density due to a poor mineral count in the bones. This eventually leads to osteoporosis which stems from breastfeeding and aluminum exposure. In addition, Respiratory Distress Syndrome also occurs due to lung immaturity. In lung immaturity, there is a preterm premature rupture of the membranes. This is where there is an induced labor due to cervical and urethra diseases. This eventually becomes enterocolitis. Enterocolitis is a disease of the bladder and liver resulting from the abuse of alcohol and or nicotine usage.

Therefore, the chain of transmission is the source of the illness. An illness becomes a disease through a pattern is life-forces and molecular energies that are then manifested by pathogens. Bronchitis, OCPD and other diseases of the respiratory system are then conclusions of torn and rotten arteries. This can be due to genetics, prenatal deficiencies and alcoholism. As previously mentioned, alcoholism causes a variety of brain dysfunctions and urethra infections. One can then become a victim of a variety of carcinogen infections. They are ovarian, of the colon, cervix and of the appendix. In this, the individual can become overwhelmed with diseases of the brain such as cerebralism and cerebration. Therefore, this leads to a variety of motor disorders, cognitive disorders as well as a substantial form of memory loss.

Drinking alcohol while pregnant cannot only harm the infant, it can the mother as well as the father. Children are born daily due to alcoholism. They are then diagnosed with a variety of mental disorders such as

1. ADHD
2. Bipolar Disorder I or II
3. Schizophrenia
4. Autism
5. OCD

6. Other behavior disorders

7. Severely Emotional Disturbed

In addition, anemic disorders can also occur. Low blood counts, dizziness and drowsiness occurs due to iron deficiency. The hemoglobin lacks energy and oxygen due to the digestive system lacking magnesium and or magnesia. The two can be used for individuals who have an irregular heartbeat, diabetes, cancers, high blood pressure, sickle-cell, respiratory disorders and dysfunctions. This then leads to a poor digestive system. The inability to digest food properly. Finally, TB, Aids and HIV are epidemics that will continue to occur in individuals with a lack of medical awareness and improper medical attention.

In addition, The Chain of Transmission leads to PMS in men as well as women. For example,

1. Anxiety

2. Depression

3. Mood Disorders

4. Irritability

5. Fatigue

6. Bloating

7. Anxiety

8. Thyroid Disorders

Therefore, psychoactive medications combined with alcohol can create an imbalanced infrastructure within one's organic, bodily, chemical and physical developmental system. Indeed, this is within everyone's human anatomy. The periodic of elements is of the Tree of Life and The Tree of Knowledge. Therefore, beware of unclean umbilical arteries as they could lead to pulmonary tuberculosis. This occurs as there is a form of poor blood and blood cells that are oxygenated from the lungs to the heart. In this, this eventually leads to an enlargement of the heart. This causes serious infection throughout the circulatory system. In addition, this causes other diseases to occur. As previously mentioned, this leads to aneurisms of the brain as well as hemorrhaging. As hemorrhaging is a discharge of blood from the blood vessels.

Hemorrhaging can cause neuropathy of the PNS, ANS and the CNS. This can also lead to epileptic seizures in early to adult stages of a newborn. This too is a result of brain damage / chronic brain dysfunction in most anemic patients. Indeed, there are alcoholic seizures resulting from binge drinking and or the consumption of alcoholic beverages. This then results in infection of the following; liver, lung, heart and brain.

In addition, portions of the cerebral cortex become infected due to a lack of oxygen and poor circulation of cell membranes along the cell walls. Emphysema and Chronic Obstructive Pulmonary Disease also occurs due to inhalation of asbestos. This also leads to mesothelioma. Mesothelioma isn't only a military it is a disease that can occur in individuals who have lived in and or around dust and fumes. The environment of which they reside or are involved has been unclean and or they have been around chronic chemical users.

This could be the medications that are causing these diseases and disorders. Chemical overdosage cause the shallow breathing syndrome. In this, chronic fatigue syndrome (CFS). Therefore, mental exertion is when an individual has lack of patience and understanding of his/her sickness, disease or disability. You see, whenever an individual lacks knowledge and understanding of self. – This leads to disease and health disorder.

Now, through spiritual development and guidance of by one's ancestors – the individual will begin to heal by the use of Eastern medicine, diet, exercise and meditation. You see, the European, Christian, Jew and Arab has not only enslaved the African, - It has enslaved its own with greed, theft and lies. Their cheating ways has been passed on from generation to generation.

You see, a tradition is a behavior and with conditions that are passed on within a group and or society with a symbolic meaning or special significance with origins of the past. In this, there is racial division that has been mentioned throughout the Book of Genesis as Canaan was to be cursed as well as when the Philistines invaded and conquered Egypt in chapter 10. This has been a chemical and substance that has fouled the nations of ancient Kemet and Canaan as well as the eternal Godhead of the Ausarian religion prior to the creation of Adam and Eve.

The African Race has been quarantined by its' captors. Therefore, this is symbolic to the sense of substance abuse as it relates to alcoholism and other forms of drug abuse. You see, the African race had been enslaved as a result of trade at the hands of illegal drugs as well as moonshine. From the house of Jacob to Rebecca and Rachel towards Joseph in Genesis / , there has been a use of pharmaceutical substance that has caused the Hebrew to hallucinate regarding their belief system as well as their heritage of which they had stolen from the people of Egypt and Canaan . Ezra 9:2 as it relates to intermarriage it says that they have taken some of their daughters as wives and their sons, and have mingled the holy race with the people around them. Similar and contrary in Surah 6:133. You were raised from the seed of other people.

Therefore, the Muslims and Israelites have been so-called informed that they are the "holy race" – "holy seed". This is a fallacy to the maximum of creation they have denounced the African nations and tribal regions throughout the entire world ever since the creation of the Hebraic doctrine was created as it relates to Genesis 10. Moving right along and back to my point! Substance abuse and mental illness has depicted the African as negative creatures since the times of Noah as well as the writing of the Holy Quran.

In this, as previously mentioned, the Holy Quran denounces drunkards. This is a practice that goes against their doctrine. However, their leaders have been known as alcoholics as well as to have filthy perversions of watching porn and molesting children. Therefore, this leads to a greater form of insubordination throughout the world of education as well as theology, medicine and healthcare. You see, mental illness is a unique way of disharmonizing humanity. It is a means of trafficking illusions and delusions into the minds of the innocent and lowly. This was written in The Metu Neter Volume 1 – By Ra Un Nefer Amen 1. This is also common sense.

Therefore, the breath of life verses the sting of death syndrome is a critical way of viewing the entire scenario of the setien. The Devil has taught you that you shall not meditate, practice yoga, have a healthy diet and not to observe his / her tactics of inconsistencies regarding the image and likeness of God. Individuals are then used as tarot cards as written in Hebrews chapter 6 and in the Quran – Surah 17:75 There is a double punishment for non-believers during and afterlife. In addition, the punishment also occurred in Genesis 30: 14-22 as the psychedelic drug - / mandrake was given to Jacob to stimulate his sexual performance prior to the birth of Joseph. The mandrake was used for magical means. In this, the mandrake alters and agonizes the SSRI's. This made Jacob love his wife Rachel more than he loved is other wife Leah. In this, there was incest, prostitution and concubinage. As Deborah was false prophetess as well as a prostitute.

You see, Jacob was born in Paddan Aram where the Canaanites were. This is now where Syria is located. Jacob was later renamed as Israel in Genesis 35:9. You see, this is a story of hatred and greed that has been induced by the biblical writers as well as the Christian, Caucasian, Greek, Hebrew and Arab. They knew and know that this is destroying the future generations of African nations as well as the Negro of all nations. You see, Judges 4 is where there is war and conflict with regards to the conquest of the {Philistines} who branched out from within the Egyptians and Canaanites.

In this, mental illness as far as substance abuse addictions have distracted and destroyed the minority. The minority who at one instance in time were the majority. You see, slavery to substances have lead the African culture into a modern form of slavery. This form of slavery is; mental slavery. In mental slavery due to substances that are induced also incorporates lies. Lies and deception about one's own culture can lead to the addiction of perverse methodologies. These methodologies and ideologies include the teachings of modern Islamic and Greek philosophies along with Christianity. Christ was born a Muslim. If anyone has studied history, ancient history as well as ancient geography, - he or she will recognize the facts that they have no great relationship with their religious deity. The deity is fabricated into a web of delusion and grandeur.

In this, mental illness has become a method of depersonalization disorders according to the Diagnostic Statistical Manual of Mental Disorders. DSM-5. This is when an individual cries wolf constantly. This is done until the individual finally becomes mentally disabled due to his or her false and misleading accusations regarding a pre-diagnosed mental or medical condition. They, the individual then becomes conditioned with patterns and combinations of a variety of defects and complexes of the brain.

You see, the brain, circulatory, CNS, PNS and ANS can only incorporate a certain amount oxygen and energy for a certain time period. However, whenever induced with negative and unwelcomed forms of stimuli such as AODA - it eventually dies. The brain becomes comatose. This then becomes developmental methods of behavioral disorder through autism, ODD and ADHD. These are also coined as Bipolar and Schizophrenia of the behavioral spectrum. These become early stages of Parkinson's, Dementia and Alzheimer's.

You see, racism is a mental illness. Utchau Metu means the weighing of words. Whatsoever a man think, he or she shall become. This is depersonalization / Derealization Disorder. The disorder is cultural related with diagnostic issues. These issues are related with religions and cultures. Therefore, in many cases they are often misdiagnosed. However, as written in DSM – V page 304; however, these individuals who intentionally induce these states tend to lose control over them and later develop a fear and aversion for related practices.

What then is Psychotherapy? It can be culturally bias due to certain factors of the spiritually ill-informed practitioner. The practitioner often has mental conditions that must be enhanced with spiritual ritual. Therefore, behavior modifications tend to only worsen the behavior of the individual who is being modified. In addition; these conditions are of autistic behaviors. Meaning, repetitious in form. Therefore, in many cases, the educator and or practitioner at often times induce these behaviors unto the individuals to whom they are educating and or attempting to care for. These are self-induced illnesses. This is intentional acts of mental and conditional behavior.

You see, throughout my entire life and dealings with people, individuals tend to be arrogant in their misunderstandings with regarding their role in the lives of the mentally ill. Meaning, arrogance factored in the lives of everyone involved in the living. Arrogance is a spiritual disorder "Narcissism" – that is a brain and disorder of derealization. This is due to episodes of grandeur and delusion. This is coined with Schizophrenia as well as Bipolar I and or II.

In these mental illnesses, the carriers are to be responsible for their actions. However, they tend to be vagabonding and scapegoating individuals. These individuals tend to believe that everyone owes them. This can be from the simple to the largest form of anything. This individual has caffeine addictions, nicotine disorders as well as other drug related addictions. Therefore, this leads to carcinogens and abnormal tremors. Tremors lead to brain damage within the SSRI's, ANS and CNS.

In this, Individuals have become untamable within the realm of their ailing mental disorders. Not to mention, ADHD is yet another disorder of the mental capacity. This disease is a result of being overly induced with combination drug treatment. In combination drug treatment there are many factors to consider. As I've mentioned in previous books, the factors shall consist of individuals – the patient – being aware of his diagnosed medical condition(s) as well as his or her prescribed medications. This will enable the patient in becoming his / her best and or worst in determining the fate of self.

Self-knowledge is important along with a non-westernized spiritual approach throughout the healing process. Also, acknowledgement of one's own illness (diagnosis) is also a key element in the healing stages of an illness and or disability. Therefore, we must maintain an understanding that religion is not spirituality. In this, we'll recognize that mental illness can be conditional racism. In conditional racisms, there are patterns of self-denial and hatred amongst a variety of racial groups and organizations. This has lead to mental slavery and cultural degradation. In cultural degradation, there are many factors that must be understood and first recognized.

The establishment of religion was created based on racism. This is also as that of The Quad, The Holy Bible and The Holy Quran mentions. However, they have been delusional in their messages towards their followers. Things – key elements have been hidden from the people. For this particular reason, there is slavery, war and idolatry. Within these idolatry's there is greed, homosexualism and poverty. In this, there has to be some wise to this notion of bigotry and hypocrisy.

Therefore, derealization disorder can be deceiving to the eye. You see, it becomes Bipolar 1 and or 2. This ranges from mild to severe episodes of delusion and grandeur. This is not far from the substance induced form of schizophrenia and anxiety. Indeed, the spirit has to be willed in order for each individual to become resurrected within his new life or as some people say "Born Again".

Wait one minute. If God foreknew you before the foundations of the world – We must first restore our divinity of and from Khamit- Canaan. This is a true form of restoration. Restoration means to go to the root of the problem. It means to restore things into their (its) original form of existence. However, in many forms of depression. There are several causes and factors. The factors included rely on environmental factors. In this, the environment of slavery can as well be of the chattel, mental and metaphysical lack thereof. Meaning, we must as well as the physician / psychiatrist understand the cultural differences as well as the varied religions of the particular culture being dealt.

However, through arrogance and revenue; racism has laid its feet upon the soil and foundation of existence. To exist, we as a whole nation must realize the conditions that have excluded all races through stereotypical forms and methodologies by irrationalizing the purpose of each individual. What I am saying is, racism has many forms as well as mental illness. Idleness is another key factor of the stereotype that has caused individuals to have subtle stages and forms of anxiety.

Therefore, if you have observed chattel slavery as well as the history of the entire world, including ancient African civilizations - / you'll come to realize and recognize that people cannot take for granted the fact that the great civilizations of Ithiopia, Khamit and Canaan have been disguised as pagan and idolatrous nations. This is written and recognized within every form of Western philosophy, science, religion, music, medicine and educational establishment. This is a substance that has been induced into the thought process of the mentally challenged African as well as Caucasian.

However, it has been made possible for the Caucasian to excel at a greater and much faster rate the African American. As written in the Bible "Canaan shall serve Japhites and Shem forever". This has given the Caucasian the upper hand on the (chain of command). Ostracism has been developed to enslave the mind of the African. Yes, imagine that you are or have been a victim kidnappings and or chattel slavery. Chapter nine in the Book of Genesis clearly explains this phenome. This is a Setianistic world of cultural affairs as mental health care has deprived the lost / blind. In many cases this is due to the individuals own form of ignorance and arrogance.

RESTORATION OF THE MIND

The mind is a terrible thing to waste. However, in most cases, there are individuals who have been ignorant due to their abuses and mishandling of drugs, alcohol and other substances. In this, everyone must gain a greater knowledge medicinal chemistry as well as themselves through the Tree of Life of ancient Khamit / Egypt. This is a spiritual system that enables mankind to resurrect it soul, spirit and entire well-being. This is done through a diligent form of diet, health and exercise.

You see, medicine, herbs and minerals differ in the chemical developmental makeup. In this, the there are various biochemical elements within the human body as well as the body of an organism(s). Indeed, chemistry is a part of creation. In creation, comes restoration of the living process. In the living process - / there is a great deal of dying of one's spirit, soul and anatomy. Yes, within combination therapy there is a great deal of dysfunctions and disorders that each individual must overcome. Mechanisms are actually triggered within the cell membranes as well as the SSRI's and neurotransmitters. These are processes of dictating and taming various treatments of chronic disorders and diseases. This may be whether viruses and or transmitted diseases and disorders.

In this, functional medicine is to assist in the findings that result in the underlying cause or causes of illness and or disease. However, it rarely does factionize within the realm of properly healing. Therefore, it is often unproven and sometimes proven as unusual methods of the healing and nurturing factor of stabilizing the patient. Although Western medicine and healthcare has often destabilized individual patients by culture. This then becomes selective racisms.

Selective Racisms are different forms of racism that is utilized for monetary value. In monetary systems, greed and aborted rights for humane liberty is then disregarded. Yet, regarded as systemic racism. The lack of knowledge leads to spiritual and mundane dysfunctions of unjust systems of organized disenfranchisement as well as chattel methods of psychological slavery. In psychological slavery, there are a varied amount of stimuli as well as the sublime methods of grandeur and delusion that lies with the spirit-man.

Therefore, the spirit-man has been disabled by the satanic system of Western civilization. The Western Civilization has enslaved all of its captors as well as visitors by deceitfulness and hypocrisy. In this, many health professionals have manipulated the mental state of their patients by giving them a greater form of disparity. In disparity, individuals have not known which direction to turn for a proper safety-net. They have been abandoned by the evilness and cunning methodologies of arrogance and insecurities.

Insecurities has lead the lowly in a greater sense of inhumane forms of depravation. In depravation, there's a greater form of shame and doubt. This makes one ponder on the fact that there are racial lines and schematic systems that evolve within the realms of health, medicine and psychiatry. You see, there are a variety of thought processes and stages that the patient will often be faced with. Remember, whatever knowledge an individual (patient) is lacking; it will eventually come to bite him or her in the butt!

You see, the mine can only endure so much stress. In this, stress is then built to cause aneurysms and of a much greater form of anxiety. In anxiety, there are phobias as well as guilt, shame and doubt. Indeed, we have to be capable of recognizing these psychological and physiological circumstances that trigger our healing process. In most cases, we are our worst enemy. We cause our own stresses and emotional anxieties by poor diet, lack of exercise and poor methods of meditational techniques.

We too, must have a greater sense of ourselves by realizing our spiritual and mental infirmities. This is done through the Tree of Life Meditation System. Within the Tree of Life Meditation System there is a system that allows man to govern and reform itself. We must learn and trust this system. Also, there has to be an understanding and knowledge that the European / Japhite and Shemite has stolen and hidden these truths for the African as well as the African American through a bevy of tactics in brainwashing. This truly includes, lynching, rape and murder.

The genetic infection of deceitfulness has been handed down through generation. These aren't curses. These are demonic and uncaring individuals who are only out to manipulate, dictate and maintain power over all of our resources from God. God has given us universal laws as well as resources that will provide a safe-haven of inner-peace and wealth for eternities. However, the Tem-Maat man has used its prideful activities to induce and teach the lowly with its western education and religion of lies for the sake of revenue and mind control manipulation.

In addition, to this mystery; / the body of an organism is extremely relevant to the fact that the human anatomy is often triggered to respond to psychotic features in Western thought. This is in opposition to the Eastern form of spirituality and metaphysical healing. In this, cells of the CNS are a respondent to all external activity. This has an effect on the immune system and peripheral nervous system. Therefore, stimuli is to somewhat a degree of eternal existence. In many cases; stimuli is linked to subliminal messages that are then linked to trigger psychotic episodes of delusion and grandeur.

Therefore, subliminal messages can have an effect on both the conscious as well as the subconscious. Therefore, to the unspiritual sahu man or woman, this is a complex situation to comprehend. In addition, the spirit is then governed by the soul. The soul is the state of being that enables mankind to recognize external triggers of the highly sophisticated though process. Indeed, our thoughts are often triggered by desires of so-called, need and want. In want, we must seek God with all of our heart. This will enable us to tame the foolish and desirous nature of the flesh / sensual sensations through thought and stimuli.

In addition, in animal toxicology, there are many forms of stimulated procedures that occur. In this, examples of electric shock and mental methods of Pavlovian studies come into formation. This is the Westernized way of institutionalizing those by continuing to inflame their minds and thought process with mental slavery and other forms of control. Whether it be in the form of miseducation, unemployment, poor healthcare and poverty. This includes poor living and sanitation conditions.

All of this leads to a mindboggling institution. This is known as The Peculiar Institution. Therefore, my friend; do not be a slave-minded individual who has been dehumanized into a realm of the demoralizing hypocrisy of a theologian, politician or conman. This is dual diagnosis of both Narcissistic Personality Disorder and Histrionic Personality Disorder seem to overlap each other by symptoms of unappreciativeness and arrogance. This also includes a higher level of wanting to be the center of attention. There is also a greater form of charm and intellect in this type of character.

This individual becomes obsessed with same-sex relationships. Although, in some cases they have a limited amount of friends of the same sex. Yet, they are very extraverted individuals who are the life of the party. Indeed this includes a pervasive form of grandiosity (fanciful behavior patterns) that are linked to Bipolar and Schizophrenia. This includes ideational forms of power, sex and love. These individuals require a great deal of admiration. This is Het Heru / Heru Tem on the Tree of Life Meditation System. Of which was created by Shechem Ur Shechem, creator of the Ausar Auset Society.

Therefore, through arrogance, we lose our understanding of who we are, where we fit and where we ought to be in life. This leads to instability and us remaining at the sahu spirit / personality. The mind is a terrible thing to waste. This occurs through a negative thought process as well as negative subtle messages that are received daily. / - Throughout our daily activities and interactions with others. In many cases, the emotions of others can trigger the mental and spiritual development of others if there is a lack of knowledge in a given area of mental and spiritual development and nurturing.

In addition, restoration is the root of healing of the mind, body and soul. This includes having the knowledge and understanding of the need to sacrifice thoughts of negativity, grandeur and delusion. In this, various episodes are coupled with emotions that are filled with anxieties of anger and irrational thinking. This leads to institutionalizing and remanufacturing ones memories of traumatic events that have hindered ones progressive state of tranquil. Therefore, in tranquil there's a greater sense of inner-peace throughout any situation. Some situations may seem horrendous to the point of malice, homicide and suicide. However, meditation is the renewing of the mind and mental / - thought process.

In mantras there is a greater sense of harmony with the individual true divine nature and self. This is not a sense of arrogance / self-rightness.

This is God's plan for all of humanity. Whereas; you were foreknown before the foundations of the world. The world is a place where the physical body resides. However, we must live in the heavenly spirit – soul and mind of inner-peace, just and unity of the spirit.

The spirit, through meditation allows the chakra of the body to be rejuvenated with opulence and greatness of the spirit. You see, meditation alters the spirit. Therefore, the hypocrisy within psychiatry, the church - / has contributed to racism, hatred and socialism. What they preach and teach are subject to manipulation of ones lower being. Ministrys exploit ones weakness and or weaknesses with the Holy Bible, Torah, Quran and Book of Mormon. This by giving motivational speeches that sooth ones emotional state for a short time period.

In this, individuals tend to have episodes of delusion and grandeur that are coupled with maniacal mood swings that often interferes with ones living conditions. In most cases, there are scoffers who observe your spiritual ritual situation and obstruct you methods. You see, scoffers are often within your spiritual real to hinder you knowledge with pleasurable and enticing dramas. These dramas include situations of likes and dislikes.

They enter you mediation and prayer life to save their asses. Have they never had Grace? Have they Fallen into the lower pit of the sahu spirit man? Therefore, surrounding youself with a positive circle of friends is must when dealt with any form of circumstance. Mentally, one must surround itself with nurturing individuals who understand and have gone through similar situations as they have in order for them to find better coping skills and the ability to maintain sanity.

This is a difficult task! However attainable. Therefore, information doesn't alter the individual's behavior. Meaning, conditions that are opposed to results of meditation. Dreams too can be altered through meditation. Obstructions can also be altered through meditation. In addition, one must show that he or she is willing to sacrifice his own will in order of pursuing and attaining a positive relationship with God through meditation. You see, there's always room for improvement of one's person as well as self.

The mind, therefore, goes through several processes. Thought goes through several process. In addition, there has to be balance within thought as well as the mind. What you are thinking can overtake you. You mental state of being is challenged daily and throughout life with worldly hopes and expectations. We can be triggered by the actions and thoughts of others if we aren't careful and lack knowledge of the Tree of Life.

This is a known fact that slavery has manipulated this world into a diagnosis of mental illnesses that are coupled with conditional behaviors that have lacked stability with episodes of torture, maiming and murder. Exodus 21:20 says that anyone that beats their male or female slave with a rod must be punished if the slave dies as a direct result. But they shall not be punished if the slave recovers after a day or two, since the slave is their property.

Now, this is a serious and sadly shameful example of modernity as it lies within reach and the outskirts of the human mind. The African mind - / The mind of the mentally ill. You see, we have to realize that slavery exists not only in the physical and spiritual. However, also within the soul and heart of every human being. This is a multitude of dire shame as it has demoralized poor communities as well as the impoverish. This has tamed the minds of the lowly. Numbers 23:9 I see a people who do not even know themselves. This is meant to say that individuals can be mentally impaired even though they haven't been touched by the slaver. This is to say that racial discriminations and allegations of brainwashing also is a part and the art of the master, pastor, preacher, bishop, prophet, evangelist, teacher and high priest.

This is a philosophical form of slavery that has existed throughout colonialism and the invasions of Khamit, Canaan and Ethiopia by the Caucasian, Jew, Arab and Christian. There is yet no understanding of this great outrage of sanctifying racism, greed, hatred and mental torture. By no means are the minds of billions to be mentally ill. However, there is a greater form of spiritual wickedness in high places. Meaning, those with wealth and leadership positions have and are in control of our thinking by the tactics of scheme.

This too is idolatry, narcissistic that leads to various individuals having histrionic personality disorder. In this, they are characterized by ignorance, arrogance and prude behaviors and uncontrolled conditions and maniacal temptations that involves cheating, stealing and denial. You see, God is unconditioned and love. The power is within you and I to delete the scars of mental genocide that was caused as a result of generational curses by the House-Nigga and

Wicked European immigrant millions of years prior. This is as Adam and Eve weren't the first two on this universe.

Therefore, let's awaken from our slumber of darkness. Meaning – BULLSHIT! Our children have been denied proper educational training and learning of independent living at the hands of the master. That is, the slave master. Therefore, suffer not children. The lies must be exposed with regards to mental illness and mental slavery. You see, we have to understand that the purpose of slavery was to incarcerate the soul of all of humanity with regards to bigotry and hypocrisy.

Lies of the educator had conditioned and controlled the cradle of civilization with its filth of deceit. Filth and deceit to the point of various forms of conduct disorders in children, teens and adults. This has been passed and handed down throughout generations. Generational community organizers and leaders have misled the people with watered down messages of healing and social welfare that has led to the murdering of millions of innocent victims.

The education system is a systematic formulation of information that has ruined the mental process of children and adults by tormenting the sekert kind of learner and has praised the so-called intellectual great with westernized forms of praise and unworthiness. This stimulated and KKK related scheme of philosophy has been proven as affective in its mainstreaming and false practices of rehabilitating the mentally ill and substance induced being by continuing to offer medications that induce and seduce individuals into lower stations of health.

In this, there are individuals who have been starving and dying for better living conditions as well as education system. However, this is merely impossible for healing due to environmental factors. Environmental factors include, stability, lack of social interaction, lack of family structure, lack of shelter, impoverish neighborhoods and communities / - villages and etc.

In non-westernized ancient traditions, children remain home with mother until the age of four. However, this differs in our current and modern day and age. You see, western civilization and education systems have failed humanity. Whereas; the exceptional learner is often overlooked due to discrimination and prejudices. Indeed, the exceptional learner must therefore, work on his or her own coping skills by developing better living conditions (environments) of circle of friends.

Truly, you lose or have no friends as you walk through your mental health journey. However, by applying self-knowledge with regards to neurocognitive disorders is applicable. In social cognition, behaviors must be acceptable with a form of modesty in dress. Therefore, a neurocognitive disorder is a disorder that affects the entire brain. Individuals are often tested with regards to nutrient and or vitamin deficiencies. This is common and has environmental triggers and factors that are relative to mental illnesses and separation anxiety.

Racism in the educational philosophy of the western civilization has and continued to manipulate and train the thought process of the non-western. However, there are has become a much higher rate of westerners who have fallen into this category by imitating the lifestyle of the African and African American. Therefore, you cannot have your cake and eat it. You see, the manipulation leads to a variety of forms of sickness, disease and disorder.

Proper education and self-knowledge are keys to restoration of cognitive development. Proper education with regards to religious affiliation, spiritual affiliation and historical references that refer to the hidden truths that have been withheld by the slaver of the pre, post and present form of colonialism will allow individuals with mental illnesses to enhance the ability to live amongst all so-called normal people.

Misleading principles in education has led to the rise in histrionic features and disorder with extreme forms of ideation and delusion. In delusion, there are forms of cognitive hallucinations that interferes with an individual's proper cognitive functioning. You see, forgetting is the number one cause of failure. In this, failures occur due to disturbances within the SSRI's, neurons and neurotransmitters. Through neurosurgery, there are several test and x-rays that are given by the neurosurgeon that observes brain cells, brain activity and stimuli of which the brain encounters.

Subtle influences that trigger physical movements and emotional responses are also called subliminal messages. These messages are called Nekhebet and Uatchet of the Khamitic spiritual system. This system was created by Ra Un Nefer Amen. He is an author and best seller of The Metu Neter. Subliminal messages intermingle with ones' life-force Ra! The Ra force enables man to recognize and control his conditions, emotional behaviors and mental / emotional attitude from negative stimuli.

Education has informed man of certain techniques in the teaching of Special and Exceptional Education. However, spiritual things must be tooled with meditation. Education is not spiritual. It is only information. Wisdom is given through meditation of tantra and mantra! The education system causes a variety of disinhibited social engagement disorders as well as separation anxieties amongst the poor within urban communities of which the impoverish dwell.

This leads to mental illness due to daily stressors as well as anxieties that cause individuals to have and maintain structured lives. This kind of individual is often secluded and or in inappropriate relationships that leads to various kinds of gay and lesbianistic relationships. This is also known as histrionic disorder.

Within histrionic disorders and anxieties there are also features of fetishistic disorders. Fetishistic Disorders relating to homosexuality as it relates to gay and lesbian issues. This is environmentally triggered as to on, with one being abused in past or present relationships. This also relates to individuals not participating in regular male female relationships as it relates to PTSD and other affiliated anxiety disorders. This also includes the vagabond who has had several sexual encounters with both sexes in order to maintain temporary living arrangements. These individuals tend to have children to in order to hide their fetishistic gay and or lesbian relationship/s. In other words, having children or a child is a cover-up in order to continue in those idolatrous activities. In this, the education system and the Bible discusses Sodom and Gomorrah as to have been abominations.

However, it doesn't mention the fact that those were once two great and powerful nations prior to the Christian, European, Arab and Jew invading ancient Khamit and Canaan. You see, Europe is and has been barbaric since the beginning of the recording of history. In this, Lesbos, which is located in Greece is too paganistic in its own rite. This also includes Transvaal which is currently under the British rule. The monarchy of these nations have done the African people a great disservice by torture and inhumane treatment.

Therefore, idolatry was and has been first practiced by the European slaver. This must be understood as it relates to mental illness. In mental illnesses and disorders some of the causes have had environmental triggers. What I am saying is that throughout chattel slavery there was inappropriate behaviors that were manifested by the captivator. Sexual prowess was common. However, the Caucasian has used and flipped the scrip as I must say. They have been the scapegoat. We have been treated as freaks in side shows.

In addition, it has been often mentioned that Adam was the first man on earth. However, individuals who have studied any form of history are aware that Zinjanthropus is the one of the first men on earth. In this, today, individuals that carry similar features to Zinjanthropus are known to have the cancerous disease called (werewolf syndrome) - / Hypertrichosis / Ambras Syndrome. This disease is an autosomal cutaneous disorder that is caused by cancers of the skin. Autosomal is any chromosome that is not a sex chromosome.

Therefore, this is where racism plays a major role in the modern world. Whereas; somatic symptom disorder is a disorder that can be caused by a substance(s) and abuses thereof; this includes various forms of anxieties and depressions regarding ones unknown health conditions. With the cost of healthcare on the rise, the westernized system has declined the minority within the African American community.

You see, psychiatrists, physicians and Egyptologist are frustrated with these findings of economical racism. In this, we must understand the aboriginal effect of the affects of the genocidal depopulationing of the originators of the universe. That is to say that The Bible and Quran were written as forms of Judaism and Zoroastarianism. This is to say that they are of the Abrahamic religious faiths. Therefore, the Caucasian is the culprit to the cultural delusion and systemic methodologies of selective racisms that has ruined the lives of the Black generations. Through ancestry, there are diseases that were invoked by the Caucasian as forms of experimentation to create higher forms of disease as well as mental stress and emotional anger amongst the African Race. This has also created a form of higher education and learning.

Therefore, psychiatry, education and religion are systemic forms of racism. Education and race through ostracism and Jim Crowism are fueled by forms of economic sanctions with no regards the African Race. Racism and false Education leads to covetous practices such as the gay rights agenda of same-sex couples performing sexual acts in front of a child or while the child is present. This began with the European ancestry. All of which leads to the psychiatric term "Histrionic Disorder". In this, Deuteronomy 28:18 and 2 Peter

2:14 mentions the fact that children will be raised as a part of the homosexual and prostitution agendas with regards to and as a result of idolatry and forms of false education at the hands of racism within the westernized religious and economic forums of nontraditional methodologies of sacred agnostic forms of European witchcraft, superstitions and substance induced mood disorders.

In this, education is a glooming topic when it comes to psychiatry as it relates to monitoring a child or the behavior of children. Therefore, it is difficult to mainstream a child who has been brought up and raised in an environment that triggers such behaviors. Indeed, a hostile environment that includes lewdness and acts of inappropriateness will hinder a child's growth and development. I too have seen this while I've been involved with the so-called church. Whereas; preachers, teachers and individuals who are choir members are or have given birth to homosexuals, committed incest and acts of child molestation.

This has hindered the progression of humanity. They preach opposite of what they allow within their living environment. Back during slavery, as well as in our current society there were and are acts of beastiality / animal-sex is referenced as zoonotic pathogens of zoonosis. These perversions have triggered into modern forms of fetishistic disorder.

You see, this is wild, crazy and scary. Whereas; the history of the African Race has been never mentioned. Whereas; whenever the Holy Bible denounces Egypt, it fails to mention that is denouncing later generations of their disobediences as they were ruled by the Arab, Greek, Roman, Christian and Jew. Genesis 10:14 as it mentions that Egypt was the father of the Kasluhites whom the Philistines came from.

The Philistines were Indo-European maritime people who invaded Egypt in the 12ᵗʰ century BC. No doubt had conquered Canaan after its invasion. As those were the creators and manipulators of vile affections and acts of idolatrous worship.

Therefore, this is hypocrisy! Education and racism has caused many children to have a variety of conduct disorders due to kleptomania and childhood maltreatment. This could be relating to family upbringing. Meaning, the child could've been neglected due to mental, spiritual and physical abused. This could be accomplished by either by as his or her sibling(s), parent(s), guardian(s) and or another perpetrator. In this, non-parental psychological abuse often occurs within ones friendship circle, spiritual or religious circle or current living situation. Whereas; mental illnesses are medical illness that often have environmental triggers.

This is generational through an individual's present, personal and past history. Whereas; anyone can be affected as the perpetrator too needs psychiatric guidance. Truly, in an unraveling sense of darkness, prostitution and substance abuse factors are due to a child transporting drugs for the pimp or pusher which leads to the involvement of the local law enforcement agency as well as child protective services. Therefore, individuals become unstable vagabonds and drifters which leads to kleptomania and opposition defiance disorder resulting from relational and grieving problems.

Inappropriate relationships tend to carry the weight of those involved by terms of sexual, physical and or psychological distress. In this, The Bible is a motivator. However, motivation and information doesn't heal or resolve the current mental condition or conditions therof. It conceals the fact that throughout history there have been kleptomaniacs and deceivers (Shemites – Japhites) who have destroyed the African race with its histrionic features of flatter and forms of delusion when it comes to the truth as it relates to unconditional love.

Special Education, religion and racism have been created by the belittling Egyptologist and White man. They have used various forms of Gay Tarot, Wicca and Gay Witchcraft to seduce the lowly. In this deception, this has created and regenerated racism, hatred and idolatry. All of which has been reformed in Europe and passed along the entire western civilization as a pit-bull for the already established demonic democracy of brainwashing and mental slavery.

In this, children are born of a curse and or curses with a variety of mental disorders. King David and Joshua were chosen and manipulated into creating wars to conquer Egypt and Canaan. The leaders of Israel used the oracle Urim Thummin which was derived from ancient Kemet in order to justify their passions and desires of invasion, conquer, rule and division. You see, in this, both King David and Joshua were youth as they were chosen to lead their particular nation – ISRAEL into battle. Also, one must take into account that in our current events in the Middle Eastern nations that was Kemet and Canaan.

Whereas; their children are forced and born into becoming active within the military. Also, as soldiers and suicide bombers. This is where mental illness is prevalent among children, youth and young adults in the western civilization. The Holy Bible and Quran are deceptive. The two are filled with lies and deceptive. As 2 Samuel 1:26 King David was gay. Therefore; this leads to a mental state of confusion as written in Deuteronomy 28:28. Whereas; the children and adults become diagnosed with a variety of mental illness as a result of the hypocrisy amongst religious leaders, Egyptologists and educators due to racially biased teachings.

Individuals are subjected into mental slavery and bigotry. Therefore, there is no forgiveness with regards to lies of hostile forms of torture by individuals who reign in high social places and political organizations. This was written in Ephesians chapter six by Apostle Paul. However, Paul lead a life too of hypocrisy. You see, the children suffer. Whereas; the consequence of the "holier than now" parent, preacher, teacher leader has convinced them into this form of behavior shaping and mainstreaming. Read 1 Samuel 20:30 and Leviticus 20:13 as they contain vile act of affection as it relates to Judaism and the House of Israel.

For these purposes, there is a constant rise in perverse, idolatry and criminal behavior amongst the lowly, the African as well as the wealthy church-going son of a bitch who has imposed its generational lies amongst the blind. This has been accomplished by manipulating an individual's lower being within the animal spirit by being judgmental against of the Tree of Life Meditation System that was created by Shechen Ur Shechem, Ra Un Nefer Amen 1. As we all know that the world has been twisted with lies and misunderstandings regarding the parables that have been written in the Holy Bible and Holy Quran. Lies pertaining to true Kemetic spiritually has smothered the human race. Whereas; many so-called scholars have false-claimed the knowledge of God, self, religion, Black Culture and race relations. This has hindered progression of the entire world and all of creation.

This becomes a battle for the mind as it relates to diagnostics and statistics regarding mental disorders and malfunctions of societal health. This becomes genocide and psychopathic racism. Whereas; psychopathology is of violence of which individuals tend to harm themselves as well as others. Racism is when individuals become obsessed with forms of hatred towards other races of people. Therefore, psychopathic forms of racism is when individuals will do whatever is vital in the causatives to harm particular groups of people. Whether it be of a different race, tribunal, religion, gender and or origin. This leads to hatred, wars and more criminal activity.

MENTAL ILLNESS DUE TO SUBSTANCE ABUSE

You see, mental illness and substance abuse can be related to a variety of medical conditions. Whereas; in ancient Egypt the Carnelian is focused on giving energy by boosting an individual's creativity and protecting one from negative emotions: It helps with digestion and menstrual cramps. The Mandagoras is a plant (drug) that grows in Jerusalem as well as Palestine. Palestine was Canaan. Therefore; seek medical assistance for dealing with health problems. Genesis 30:14-21 in the story of Jacob, Rachel, Rebekah and Leah it discusses the sexual relations as well as the substance induced mood disorders that had occurred as a result of its intake.

This is similar to what goes on in our current day. Sin is an abomination and antipsychotic and antidepressants tend to cause panic and anxiety disorders. In most psychiatric drugs there is a slow-kill syndrome attached to their triggers. As the majority of medications aren't for the benefit of the African Americans. There is a probationary period for damaging symptoms to occur.

In this, there are various forms of abuse of substances that tend to cause depressions, anxieties, cancers, aids, HPV, HIV and other venereal diseases. For example, nicotine addiction is prevalent amongst individuals with mental illnesses, such as anxiety, bipolar mania, schizophrenia and or major depression disorder. Individuals often get SIDS, heart disease, asthma, hepatitis, COPD and or bronchitis as a result of nicotine addiction. In this, nicotine is created from the tobacco plant (Nicotiana Tabacum) which is found in foreign countries. Such as South America, The Bahamas, Eastern Eurasia and parts of Africa and Australia. Individuals are victims of a genocidal epidemic as a result of attaining PTSD after the Mid Atlantic Slave Trade and or serving in the military where Green Tobacco Sickness (GTS) was formed.

(GTS) causes nausea, vomiting, headache, dizziness and severe weakness in locomotion processes with regards to the mammalian and limbic system of the brain due to damaged motor neurons. Note: in tobacco leaf exposer there is an increase within depression and comatose rates. This also includes neuromuscular blockades, blood disease, discomfort and constant urination, Blood in urine, epileptic seizures, CNS infection with tremors, muscular weakness and diseases, autoimmune and skeletal diseases, respiratory paralysis due to destroyed dopamine inhibitors, SSRI's and neurotransmitters.

In addition, (GTS) causes hepatitis, constipation, hypertension, epilepsy, sexual dysfunction or increased sex drive which causes various sexually transmitted diseases. This also causes delayed speech or increased speech patterns as nicotine receptors are ruined as a result of an antidepressant effect. It also causes various forms of mild to major depressive disorders that includes bipolar, anxiety and schizophrenia as one become behavior addiction compulsive due to nicotine addiction.

As previously mentioned, mental illnesses are of various medical illnesses that have environmental triggers. As from an addictive personality disorder one becomes emotionally insecure with separation and or attachment disorders resulting for narcissistic and histrionic behavior patterns. As far as Addictive Personality is concerned, this deals with the following; isolation from others, antisocialism and the inability to deal with stressful situations. In addition, this is the lower level of the Kemetic Tree of Life. The sahu division.

Addictive Personality is within one who will lie, cheat, steal and murder. Those acts are done in order to preserve the addiction. Aggression is greater than the typical behavior. This also includes histrionic mood disorders of fraud and identity theft along with writing bad checks and looting. Also in addiction, there is an interruption within the mammalian, reptillian and cerebral cortex of the brain. By these areas being endangered, harmed and or undeveloped, this causes negative conditioned behavior patterns of various forms of addiction. Such as sexual, substance and idolatry.

Moving right along, the following serve as antidepressants as well as stimulants that will eventually destroy the arteries as well as the brain. They are slow-kill street drugs are illegal in many states:

1. Cannabis
2. Cocaine
3. Chrystal-Meth
4. Heroine

Caffeine too is a stimulant that can cause sleep deprivation. It is also used as an antidepressant and mood stabilizer. Medical and psychological problems occur when using caffeine. They are; Memory loss, difficulty thinking, constant urination, anxiety, depression and insomnia.

1. Memory loss
2. Difficult thinking
3. Constant urination
4. Anxiety
5. Depression
6. Insomnia

These are genetic disorders that are shared with cigarette smoking and alcohol which are similar in their effect. Individuals who are in use of caffeine have generalized anxiety disorders and panic attacks due to a lack of patience and or holistic understanding as it relates to anything.

In addition to this, Oxycodone and Eukodal are also addictive. Oxycodone is an addictive medication that is used by all races and genders. However, African American females are most likely to become addicted says the American Psychological Association. Oxycodone also produces suicidal tendencies and are used as stimulants and antidepressants. Individuals often have cravings for this drug similar to mandrake of The Holy Bible in Genesis!

This particular drug, Oxycodone causes memory loss and ruins the central nervous system, ANS and PNS. It causes respiratory failure and respiratory depression. In addition, it causes, upper respiratory infections. Such as lung, liver cancer and heart disease. You see, in nursing mothers the use of oxycodone causes miscarriages, abortions, cancers of the ovaries, cervix, gastrointestinal and uterine. However, in men and women, it causes prostate cancers as well as thyroid cancer. Cancerous blood is found in African Americans. However, in all races myopathy (weakness in muscles) occur along with liver disease and jaundice (yellowish skin).

Also, in Oxycodone addiction as muscle relaxants, it causes hepatitis, depression, high blood pressure, constipation and mental confusion. In this, children are born deformed and or mentally retarded. This is similar to morphine. Morphine is another drug that can easily be addictive as a pain reliever in adults as well as children. It causes the following:

1. PTSD
2. Bipolar – Euphoria – Elation
3. Schizophrenia

4. Idleness

5. Borderline Personality Disorders

6. Major Depressive Disorder

7. Loss of cognitive control

8. Impaired judgement

9. Cancer

In addictive personality, individuals will do whatever is necessary in order to get illegal and over the counter drugs. These are slow-kill pharmaceuticals as is cancerous meats. For example, chicken, pork, turkey and beef contains various carcinogens of arsenic. The arsenic can also cause diseases in arteries, diabetes, heart disease, anxiety and thyroid diseases.

Whereas; these foods were leftovers that were given by slave masters during slavery. Currently, they are being injected and contaminated with steroids and bulked as infants and sold prematurely for retail. This is known as Fowl Cholera. During the ancient of days, The African was vegetarian prior to being invaded, conquered and enslaved by the slaver.

REPROBATED MINDS

Leviticus 18:22-23 man do not have sexual relations with a man as one has with a woman, that is detestable. Do not defile yourself to have sexual relations with an animal. A man or woman must not present themselves to an animal to have sexual relations with it. This is perversion. Leviticus 20:13 they shall be put to death. In addition, Romans 1: 26 - 31

Therefore, the word reprobate means unacceptable towards humanity. In addition, homosexuality, lesbianism, heterosexualism, bisexualism and beastiality are all acts of abomination. In this, men and women may possibly have more or less X and or Y chromosomes. This is through genetics and heredity. Also, note the fact that there are spiritual infirmities as an individual has a low cognitive intake of his or her own reptilian and mammalian brain potential of eliminating such activities from his or her lifestyle. This is where there is an imbalance of progesterone, estrogen and androgens. This causes sexual dysfunction.

In addition, in beastiality, penile cancer occurs in men while on the other hand, ovarian and uterine cancer in women. You see, polycystic ovary syndrome occurs as a form of amenorrhea. Amenorrhea is when an individual is obese around the abdomen.

Individuals can also be infected with White Gene Drosophila Melanogaster. In this, insect bites can also cause STD's.

In bisexual male rats the suprachiasmatic nucleus (SCN) serum is given to determine the vasopressin (AVP) neurons in heterosexual men. This is where the mammalian brain levels are high in levels of estrogen. This becomes Hypoactive Sexual Desire Disorder. This also becomes sexual selection disorder of sexual dimorphism. Whereas; within the hypothalamus there is a dysfunction. This is linked to the pituitary gland, CNS and endocrine system. This causes immunological diseases as well as sleep disorders.

Mental illness is of many medical conditions that have environmental triggers. Ephesians chapter 6, in many cases, this is spiritual wickedness in high places. King Herod's are everywhere. There are gay and lesbian dream spells that are invoked through forms of Wicca and maniacal methods of racist theology and philosophy. In this, substance medication induced sleep disorders can be due to other mental or medical illnesses. These illnesses include,

(a.) Insomnia Disorder
(b.) Parasomnia
(c.) Hypersomnia

Those disorders are stemming with the following disabilities and or illnesses:

1. Mental Disorders
2. Bipolar Disorder
3. Schizophrenia
4. Anxiety
5. Substance use disorders
6. Cannabis
7. Ecstasy
8. Early stages of Dementia
9. Diabetes
10. Cancer
11. Hepatitis
12. Parkinson Disease
13. Anemia
14. Maple Syrup Urine Disease
15. Narcolepsy

Whereas; parasomnia is when there are abnormal movements, behaviors, emotions, perceptions and dreams that occur during and between sleep stages. In this, an individual's Chromosome 6 Genes are damaged leading to the above. In other words, Hypersomnia is when there is an excessive form of daytime sleepiness due to one or all of the following; head trauma, epilepsy, autoimmune thyroiditis, lupus, nephritis, autoimmune hepatitis, liver inflammation and jaundice. This also includes damaged tissues and nerves within the CNS, PNS and ANS.

In addition, it is written and mentioned by various psychiatrist and physicians have mentioned that African Americans have cirrhosis of the liver due to prescription drug abuse, drug abuse and alcohol abuse.

Shame on all physicians. For they are reprobated. For they have written prescriptions for painkillers, penicillin (antibiotics) and sleep aids such as; Ertatenen, Vancomycin, Sluconavole, Oxycodone, Zaleplon and Zolpidem. These medications are of genocide towards the lowly (blind) and the African American Community; in this, all of them cause several neurological and problems of all arteries. In addition, they cause sickle cell anemia, iron deficiency anemia, pernicious anemia and leukemia.

You see, there are several diseases and disorders that are obtained and triggered from pain killers, sleep aids and various forms of penicillin. Colon cancer, damaged arteries, respiratory infections and Red Man Syndrome with rashes. All of which leads to HIV and other venereal diseases.

In Zaleplon and Zolpidem individuals tend to have symptoms of sedative hypnosis, auditory and visual hallucinations, depressions and confusion. They also have mood swings and episodes of delusion and grandeur. This also includes night sweats, seizures, vomiting, muscle cramps and convulsions. In addition, they have effected coordination, constipation, diarrhea, muscle aches laziness and hepatitis.

The slaver injected and sedated its slave with doses of hallucinative and mood altering drugs such as medroxyprogesterone acetate and doxepin to maintain control over them as if they were animals who were distempered. Therefore, the reprobate is a racist and bigot. Romans 1:25 They have changed the truth into lies and have worshipped various forms of distractive and obstructive forms of paganism in order to seduce the African into a life of substance induced methodologies that has caused harm to trillions of innocent victims throughout several generations.

In this, the Holy Bible mentions that the Canaanites will serve Shem and Japheth. This means forever. In addition, it promises a savior for all of mankind. This is a fable. Therefore, we cannot be redeemed by Judaism and Greek philosophers. This is racism, denial and undercover hatred. You see, we cannot be pleased with a rapid form of systemic hatred and racism through western philosophy and theology. This the exact thing that put us in the condition that we are currently living in throughout this generation.

You see, they follow you. However; they follow the opposite of what you follow. They worship the creature instead of the creator. That's racism. Genesis 10:14

Mentions that Egypt was the father of the inhabitants of upper Egypt: The Pathrusites – Caphtorites of Crete, who were in ancient times residing as the Philistines. The Philistines were indo-European people who invaded Egypt and later conquered and settled in Canaan.

The Philistines were Caucasian. Enthusiastic children were brainwashed into going into battle for the sake of racism and the setien. Moses, King David and Joshua -----------They were deceived and promised kingdoms of riches and righteousness. Today, children are deceived into believing in pagan holiday. Such as Thanksgiving, Halloween, Christmas and Easter.

You see, individuals have followed the traditions of men since the Greek philosophers had found the truth was in Kemet and Canaan. Galatians 1:14 Paul writes that he was advancing in Judaism at an early age. He mentions that he was more gifted than those who were his own age as well as the elders.

You see, as he advanced in Judaism he used trickery on others. 2 Corinthians 12:16 I caught you by craftiness of the false forms of tithings and offerings as did he when he was King Saul. You see, Corinth and Gaul are in Greece. Therefore, we have been bewitched by the European lie of the savior of Judaism. Lies have been conceptualized as racism has increased while genocide amongst the African continent has plagued the African American residing in our modern civilization. Lies, hypocrisy and trickery is what brought the African into chattel slavery. Indeed, mental slavery as well as several forms of mental illness / diseases.

Whereas; it was Judaism, Islam and Christianity that has perpetrated its hand on the Egyptian, Canaanite and Ethiopian. This is a form of great depression that lies within The Jesness Inventory - 1962-1996 where individuals have been diagnosed with withdrawal depression as well as cultural conformity disorder. Biblical racism has hit the world in an explosive way. It has caused a variety of enslaved, hospitalized and incarcerated individuals to fall victim to the mainstream mechanisms of colonialized hatred at the hands of the setien.

LDS missionaries followed the pursuit of western states that are within the United States of American along with South America and Carib nations throughout the 18ᵗʰ and 19ᵗʰ centuries as we know of today. You see, it is the mission of the missionary to sway the weak into their faith as they preach and teach restoration of the church and the resurrection of Christ. Whereas; LDS doesn't inform its elders of its origin and how it became Mormon. You see, the suffix of Mormon comes from the Egyptian root Mon / which equates to Amen / Amen Rah in the Egyptian Hieroglyphic Dictionary according to Egyptologist, E.A Wallis Budge.

Also, one must note the facts that are written in the Commentary volumes of the LDS by George Reynolds and Janne M Sjodahl of it being represented as contrary to what is written within the Biblical Quad. The Quad is a book that contains the Holy Bible and yet it too has other books that so-called inspired Joseph Smith to create through several revelations the he had received from God, the Holy-Spirit and Christ.

You see, this is a non-mysterical truth. They've covered their rear ends to the point where they train the youth into becoming missionaries to a religious faith that has murdered African American – Buffalo Soldiers, Hispanics and various Indian tribal nations for the sake of Joseph Smith. What they fail to mention is that Joseph Smith too studied Judaism, The Caballah and the Illuminati. Smith tells his followers that they must become martyr's of the Mormon faith as does Islam. D&C 103:27 Saints are required to give their lives in defense of truth. Let no man be afraid to lay down his life for my sake; for whoso lay down his life for my sake shall find it again. This is taken from Luke 14:33 and Matthew 10:39.

You see, these Caucasians were and are consistently delusional. Whereas; they were full of deceptions that inspired Christendom to the form of forbidding the spiritual practices and of the African ritual. In this, The Arab and White Man are all over the Holy Bible. For this purpose, the African American ancestry has faced turmoil at the hands of the Shemite and Japhite for generations. / - as well as generations to come. Therefore, it will only worsen as there has been slavery unto mass incarceration that his infected the Black / Negroid since meeting the Caucasian in his origin.

We have been plagued with heredofamilial diseases that has inflicted many according to a hereditary basis. This is where there are ancestral and spiritual defects occur as a result of immortal lies regarding the highly educational verses the spirited. You see, the spirited has experienced the manifestation of spiritual things verses the intellectual being informed as western education and thought has rationalized through syllogism.

In westernized thought there are methods of training and conditioning one's mind through immortal fallacies and theorizing his or her conditions and behavior patterns. Through immaturity levels as well as levels of maturity. Spiritual maturity is the understanding of the spiritual. This is when the individual sees that all things are spiritual. Understanding that spiritual things aren't necessarily done through the physical and or sensual behavioral patterns. This is to say that there is such a phrase called "Immature Conformist". In this, people have difficulties adapting to people or things. This eventually leads to adjustment and conduct disorders by children as well as teen adolescents while they are in elementary through the college levels of adulthood. Or even beyond the collegiate level of age. Which often leads to conduct disorders as well as oppositional defiance disorders due to substance abuse stemming from prenatal birth defects and heredity.

Proverbs 22:6 train up a child the way he should go and he will not depart from it. In operant conditioning there is an integration of positive and negative conditions in the behaviors of humans, animals and living organisms. This can occur in and amongst prison inmates, mental health, peers and circle of friends. Also, within the operant conditioning chamber as observed; pigeons and rats through teratology and animal toxicology "trained" individuals are only trained and allowed to do what the practitioner only allows. Therefore, they observe you as stimuli; (BAIT) and blackmail by bigots and racists as they reinforce stimuli regarding your knowledge through their cunning methodologies of ministry, education and dictation.

This is where is GLBT is observed in the Quran 4:20-21, 11:78-81 and 26:162-168 as it discusses Lot's people being tempted by men of Sodom. This is also a fact that the prohibition of homosexuality is prevalent amongst Muslims, Jew of Judaism as well as Christendom. However, it is non-sanctioned by within The United States of America and our modern day Pope. Therefore, bishops and rabbis often gave infants oral sex in their birth ceremonial rituals for hundreds of years.

In addition, as children are trained at an early age, they fail in their conditioning due GLBT being observed evidently by themselves as subliminal messages have environmental triggers. These triggers are invoked while they are sleeping. During their dream state they are unaware of what their peers and or parents are involved in. You see, perversions of sexual activities are taking place while the children are given rewards of good behavior. This too is a form of operant conditioning by the seductive setien.

The GLBTQ according to the COR Child Observation Record (1992) which studies the child's interests, development and learning abilities has been used to do just that. However, scoffers are and can be neighbors who are living the lifestyle of GLBTQ and are involved in lustful acts of perversions of the Old and New Testament customs. Homosexual is immortal. Individuals have disabilities that are caused by homosexuality and racist rants of a somnophillia. They molest you while you are asleep within the ranges of the McCarthy Scale. This test was created in 1972 with age ranges of 2.5 – 9. These are scales of children's abilities where they have followed the traditions of their European ancestors of paganism and idolatry. Whereas; there are test given to assess the mode of the fathers Gal 1:14, Timothy 3:5 combined are hellacious within itself.

Homosexuality within the home is inherited and coupled with bipolar and major depressive disorder due to ketamine abuse and other neurological disorders of the central nervous system. Homosexuality is a mental illness as well as a sexual orientation disorder.

Therefore, children are imitators and observers of their external living environment. They are born with very receptive neurons and brain cells. In this, they - / the children often become products of their environment. Whereas; mental illness is of several medical conditions that have environmental triggers. So, children become whatever their surroundings produce in most cases. If they are surrounded by perverse activities such as, GLBTQ they tend to become involved in inappropriate behavioral activities such as perversions, alcohol – substance abuse and or are products within the environment of either the criminal justice system or even institutionalized within mental institutions.

In most cases, individuals become extremely maniacal with suicidal tendencies and thought processes. They are suicidal like those who are abusing MUSTARD AGENTS in support of Isis against the Kurdish Rebels. In this, the gustatory system of which is the system of the sense of taste. Therefore, this leads to addictions, passions, lusts, cravings and desires of the animal spirit of the principals of neuroscience and Khaibit being. Indeed, the hippocampus / reptilian portion of the brain is manipulated by sublime forms of receptivity.

Sweet taste and desirous signals of urges of sensuous passions that are desirous to the human development is in need of spiritual and meditative nurturing. In many cases, certain cultures and races / nationalities have been brainwashed into bigotry, greed and pleasurable desires that interfere with their divinity. This often leads to diseases that are of the venereal as molecular energies and hemoglobic antibodies travel and trigger into an individual's bloodstream. In addition, there are critical molecules that hence the pleasurable response to the presence of certain parts of the brain and within open areas of the human anatomy.

All of which has led to cultural forms of diabetes, sickle cell anemia, perversions of lust, epilepsy and birth defects. You see sensory receptors are structures of the body which change from one energy to another. Therefore, energies can vary as they come into contact with other life-forces of electromagnetic life. This is to say, "living organism" that is has its establishment within the universal laws of God.

Discrimination and Broca's areas of the Brain leads to one's ability to discriminate taste patterns of a particular product of food. However, there is more to this subject at hand. Chemoreception and the power of the tongue are relevant within the schemes. However, the cerebral cortex dictates the lower portions of the brain as we deal with difficulties of the externalized houses of difficulties that we are faced with on a daily basis. In this, the segregative Westerner of the Khiabit - Sahu man has taken over the world of the setien with his / her scheming tactics of manipulating the lower being of others without them even being aware of the manifestation of the will – meditation and the spirit.

In addition, in many cases, there is an imbalance within the entire system of the brain. Whereas; there must be intervention. Intervention, not only with psychotropic and anti-depressants as well as anti-anxiety, parkinson's, alzheimer's and dementia medications. This is to say that the entire neurological system must be enhanced with ritual, exercise, prayer and meditation. However, so many of us has are racist through segregative thought and high narcissistic - / histrionic behavior patterns and emotions.

3 Nephi 6:15 who were the Ausarians: Now, the cause of this iniquity of the people was this_ Satan - / Setien had great power unto the stirring up the people to do all of the manner of iniquity, and puffing them up with methodologies and ideologies of homosexuality and idolatry as well as paganistic perversions and prideful thinking. Tempting them to seek for power, glory, riches and things of the world. For they are seductive spirits that seek to endeavor amongst the lowly. That is the African and African American as to having them believe that they are worthless beasts. For they have eaten the entire nervous system of the Black and minority as did Dracula.

Indeed, there is racism in education, religion, spirituality, health, medicine, psychiatry and neurology that eventually leads to total chaos. Such as; the promotion of GLBTQ. This becomes and is all made up of the mental state of which individual have been in denial for centuries till this modern day culture of "Everything is Legal" status.

Therefore, the power of the tongue within the weighing of words {"Utchau Metu"} of the Broca's portion of the brain which regulates tastes, passions and desires has ties within the reptilian and limbic systems. All of which has been misinterpreted and often misunderstood by scholars and the setien. Therefore; within the Christianized Holy Bible: Romans 4:17 The God who gives life to the dead and calls things into being that were not.

This is a key issue of the tongue. In addition; if there's no knowledge with regards to the underlying problems of psychosis as well as spiritual things, how then can we be cured of such diseases of the brain? In this, foolish things are used to confound the wise. Make note of the facts that:

1. AUTOSOMAL NERVOUS SYSTEM
2. PERIPHREAL NERVOUS SYSTEM
3. CENTRAL NERVOUS SYSTEM

Are all areas of the nervous system are intertwined to regulate each other. Therefore, is an individual is induced with alcohol or other induced drugs that cause psychosis? Truly, this will indeed harm other areas within the entire nervous system. There are then problems within certain areas of the brain, if not the entire brain.

You see, the Broca's is as previously mentioned, the portion of the brain that induces the sense of taste, cravings, passions and desires. Therefore, pathoclisis is a mechanism towards particular toxin(s) with them having the tendency to attack certain organs. Those organs then enter the DNA / RNA. This then becomes a system of contagious nerve cells within the molecular pathogens of the brain. Whereas nerve cells are in constant destruction with their abilities being decreased.

In addition, healthy nerve cells die and give birth to other forms of both the DNA and RNA. In this, there is an infrastructure of the creation of other nuclei, additional cells, molecules, atoms, protons, neurons and electrolytes that are in most cases; unhealthy strands of all forms molecular genotype. Sexually Transmitted Diseases and other diseases of the brain occur as a result of any form of craving something mentally. Thoughts are then put into action without spiritual intervention and meditation.

As far as drug diffusion is concern, addiction is extreme amongst individuals who have tendencies of easily being swayed and have low forms of esteem. In this, there is a much greater tendency of being diagnosed with a psychiatric disorder as well as MDD. They claim that western thought is the only cure of addictions and internal medical conditions. As did the Greek, Judaism / Islam, LDS, SDA, Jehovah's Witnesses and so-called Christian who forgives homosexual behavior. Jeremiah 15:6 I am weary with repentance!

Moving right along. In Phantosmia, there are a variety of forms of hallucination. A hallucination is the sensory of something that is not there on the basis of the non-realistic. This is often misinterpreted by a physical stimulus. These then creates forms of segregative and paranoid patterns of thought and syllogisms within an individual. This is known as the spirit of the Khaibit. The Khaibit is the oldest part of the spirit. This is known as the Sahu-man. Due to his to its prowess of emotions, passions and desires. See the Metu Neter Volume 1 - / page 190.

Its causes can range from head trauma to prenatal deficiencies, birth defects, nicotine addiction, alcoholism and drug abuse by either of the parents prior to creating the offspring. Phantosomia is co-existent with various psychiatric disorders. They include

Schizophrenia, MDD, Bipolar, epilepsy and alcohol psychosis. This eventually leads to Parkinson's disease and extreme migraines. Therefore, in Blood-Brain Barrier (BBB) there is a circulation of blood from the brain intracellular fluid in the central nervous system that in most cases can cause other pathogens of disease and illnesses to occur within the prion family.

Prion diseases are viral infections that can cause sleeping diseases as well as MS, congenital heart disease, COPD, diabetes, lupus, rabies, HPV, HIV, Rabies and Cerebral edema. Cerebral edema is a variety of seizure type traumas within ranges of drug addiction, sickle cell anemia and epilepsy. Therefore, the brain, therefore isn't getting enough oxygen due to improper diet and lack of cardiovascular exercise as well as meditation.

see notes,,,,,,,,,

NEUROSPINAL SYPHILLIS

Neurosyphilis is an infection of the brain and the spinal cord that is caused by the spirochete Trepoenema pallidum. The Trepoenema pallidum is where there are coiled corkscrew shaped cells that eventually spread throughout the CNS until they become visual outside the body. This is due to extreme forms of human contact. This contact can occur the saliva glands, blood pathogens and various sexual partners. Also, the practicing of poor personal hygiene can lead to viral diseases and infections.

In many cases the human skull can be damaged due to stages of neurosyphilis. In this, congenital syphilis and other infectious diseases can occur within the body of an unborn child. This is when there are lingering hereditary diseases occur. You see, neuro-spinal diseases and disorders also occur as a result of inflammation within various portions of the brain. In brain injuries, there are deficiencies due to improper diet as well as drug use and abuse to other substances.

This includes medication withdrawal and substance induced psychosis. Deuteronomy 28:27 The Lord will strike you with wasting disease, with fever and inflammation until you perish with festering sores, itch and tumors. You will not be cured.

In this, there are a variety of symptoms that usually occur. They are as follows;

A: Confusion and agitation
B: Anxiety
C: Major Depressive Disorder
D: Migraine
E: Loss of memory
F: Bipolar
G: Schizophrenia
H: Peripheral Artery Disease
I: Epileptic Seizures

Surah 6:160a they are killing children and people foolishly without knowledge of anything. For, there wisdom is foolish. God uses the foolish things to confound the wise. This is due to generational curses and plagues that the Philistines received upon themselves as a result of conquering and settling in ancient Egypt and the nations of Canaan who held the Promise Land were seven in number, are as follows:

1. Canaanites
2. Hittites
3. Hivites
4. Perrizites

5. Girgashites
6. Amorites
7. Jubusites

You see, Kenaanim were the Canaanites who were one of the seven nations of Canaan before the arrival of the conquering Israelites. Jeremiah 15:6 I am weary with repenting. In this, there is an important message. Jehovah speaks to Jeremiah. Jehovah was the God of the Jews / Hebrews. Make note: That in the Quranic Surah 17:3-4 the offspring that we bore Noah. Surely he was a grateful servant. And we made known to the Children of Israel in the Book: Certainly you will make mischief in the land twice, and behave insolently with mighty arrogance.

That is the message that The Prophet Muhammad received for his God Allah that has spread to the Muslim religion. There indeed is a conflict of interest Surah 17:75 then we made thee taste a double (punishment) in life and a double (punishment) after death, and though wouldst not have found a helper against Us.

Education! Racism

****** God is,,,,,,,,

FALLEN FROM GRACE

LDS is a religious group of mercenaries and slavers too. They were mariners. In addition: Alma 41:4 and if their works are evil they shall be restored unto them evil. Therefore, all things shall be restored to their proper frame____ mortalitiy raised to immortality, corruption to incorruption. See Surah 17:75.

Alma 38:38 mentions __ and now my son, I have somethings to say concerning the thing which our fathers call a ball, or director---our our fathers called it Liahona - Annu - which is being interpreted, a compass; and the Lord Prepared it {Their god prepared it, ways of traveling and navigating new lands for slave trade and idolatrious passions}.

In addition, The base word Annu-in Liah-ona means Ra - Life-force and God in Khamit and the Cosmological priesthood of the V Dynasty of (Heliopolis). This is within the Heka and origin of the spheres on the Tree of Life initiation and spiritual system of the Ancient Egyptians and people of Canaan. This is of the Ausarian religion which goes back over 10,000 years BCE. In this, the male side of Seker rules over the death process and continues to judge the dead within their existence of not living in harmony with the laws of Maat.

Metu Neter Volume I page 222

Therefore; grace is forgiveness, understanding and love. However, when will Africa, Egypt / Canaan be restored. The restoration of ancient Egypt / Canaan is vital for the sake of humanity. For thousands of years the world has been disabled with infirmities of mental illness. This due to the untold truths regarding Africa, ancient Khamit and Canaan. You see, to restore something is it return it to its proper destination of strength and fruitfulness. However, the Caucasian has lied about a Christ who is of the European stature. Yet, has denounced the facts of the African Spiritual systems of the ancients and has crippled humanity with lies regarding a white saviour. Such as the AME church terrorist who murdered nine innocent victims!

The Bible and other religious books were written to enslave the true African mentally. This has been a success for years until the future of the 21st century. In addition, mankind has believed the lies due to its ignorance of dignity and lack of self-reliance. Therefore, biblical writers have disguised themselves as scholars for and of humanity. They have deceived the world into having them believe that such things will heal the nature of humanity. Indeed, there must be a stopage of filthy lies through misleading religious leaders and the church.

The contrawise Bible, Quran and Book of Mormon had been written as a way of enslavement. In enslavement, you get torture and brutality of the mind, body, soul and spirit. Note, this message is a valid message that will insure equality for all. All have come to know jesus christ as their saviour. I haven't. For I know that there were individuals who performed much greater works than he could have ever imagined.

Indeed, Sound Doctrine isn't that of Christianity as mentioned in 2 Timothy 4:3-5. Christianity has enslaved the souls of Black Folk. The African has been in captivity by the heathanistic slaver and historical bigot through capitalism and colonialism. Therefore, bigots cannot be bigots. Hebrews 6 has denounced the Christ within its commentary. In so on, The Israelites of The Holy Quran also denotes the Hebrew as criminal and dishonest. Alma's commentary of the Book of Mormon also understands and explains that restoration existed hundreds of years prior to the Israelites being given the title of the so-called the chosen people.

In addition; all have fallen. Lets look at the biblical context on grace and fallen. Lets look at how it describes that:

Fallen from grace Galatian 5: 1-5. By your own works and works of the law has led millions of individuals into darkness and temptations from Hell. Is it that Christ has become no affect unto you as you continue to be justified by evil deeds of willful ignorance and idolatry. Romans 6:2. Many have fallen from grace due to the inability to understand that redemption only occurs to those who have totally stopped sinning. So, what then does grace mean as well as sin and fallen.

Idolatry is a great amount of sin. This means worshipping an athlete, man or woman. Worshipping idols and loving anything more the love of the Lord. This also includes acts of prostitution and homosexuality. This includes all for which is similar to chapter I in Romans, where same sex unions and ungodliness occurs. These methods of religious practices go beyond Christianity. -Ayah 54 surah condemns these things that the church has failed to preach regarding humanity.

In the 57th Surah of the Quran it discusses the fact that during Islamic daughters time of Lot where men refused to take women as wives. They were pleased with anal intercourse and pagan worship. The church leaders preach man-pleasing sermons for only offerings and tithes. Money under the table as; money-laundering.

What then is sin? Why do we continue in sin? We are fallen people like the Adamites It is the lukewarm ministers who cause divisions within the church. These ministry's go as far as they can to divide and conquer both the single and the married. This is by the uses and practicing of idolatry. By all means, they use a variety of oracles that are varied in culture. Cults are mainly accepted within the church. Yet, un-recognized by its members. We are fallen from grace and continue to live in sin. If Christ be the people and the people are the church as the scripture says, why is grace abound?

The definition of sin is an act that violates God's Wil. It also means a Transgression of God's Divine Law. A willful act to violate orders of a God. Also, religious orders and biblical principles that are written in scriptures.

Mankind has no understanding of sin, fallen and grace. Sin is complex. In as much, as to the will of man. Man's understanding has been limited to simple addition. An inability to connect the dots. You see, the fall of Set of the Ausarian religion as well as the fall of Adam the Old Testament. This is of course from a theological prospective. It is difficult to withstand temptation and sin unless you have been educated on its surface. Its surface is of the demonic realm. The demonic realm is a spirit that dwells in the earth, soul and heart of man. Whatsoever a man thinketh he is he or she shall become. However, mans imagination is controlled be the desires of lust, perversion and idolatry. The left side of the brain is controlled by ones thought patterns.

In many cases, sin is pre-ordained by others unknowingly. This is through a form of witchcraft and or ones abuse of his or her psychic abilities. /this is often used against the will the victim. Judas is a prime example of man's jealousy against his brethren. As grace is divine favor and goodness with great will. It was Judas who betrayed Jesus many times. Man's sensitivity is badgered and taken for granted by the spiritual realm. When walking in the spiritual it is difficult to please others. You'll be often hated and or ignored by others and left as a loner or outcast to society.

Didn't Jesus Christ say, "If You Love Me They Will Hate You". For this purpose, man has fallen into temptation and the snare of the Devil. On the otherhand, psychiatry is used by the noncertified. They would rather use and oracle or tarot card to identify with those particular spirits and or emotions. This is of themselves and others. Deuteronomy 18:10-11 There shall be no one of you who makes his sons or daughters walk through fire, or useth divination or witchcraft, or an observer of time, or an enchanter or a witch. Or a charmer with familiar spirits.. Where is grace! Is grace given unto those live by the law and oracle of {Tehuti/Maat} ?

Sin is of the flesh. Flesh must die from sin so the spirit be refreshed daily. When the spirit is refreshed daily sin will not prevail against the soul of which it came. Within the spirit, spirits attempt to tempt the flesh. This is where drug addictions, perversions and idolatry occur. Your flesh is limited and the spirit is also limited. One must first die to the flesh and open to awaken the spirit.

Whenever one has fallen from grace, one becomes addicted to his or her sin. That sin can be liquor, crack-cocaine, marijuana and fornication. Fornication is sex without being married. This becomes adultery. This leads to stealing, gambling, denial and lying. This is an act of one being institutionalized in a healthcare facility or prison. In many cases, those are the two places where they would rather be.

We have fallen from grace like the demons who had been cast into the swine in the Gospels. Whereas, members of the occult wage war by spying out the liberty of Christianity. Galations 2:4 And that because of false brethren unawares brought in, who came in privily to spy out our liberty that we have in Christ Jesus, that they might bring us into bondage; Philippians 2:12 but in my absence, work out your own salvation with fear and trembling.

Those two verses are powerful in their interpretation. This is due to the fact that false brethren attempts to work out their own salvation in your absence with schemes of satanic treachery. That's one of the reasons why we are fallen from grace.

Israel was in constant instability with God during the old testament times and was often forgiven. Therefore, judgment must come upon those who are fallen. The fallen have shown a lack of reverence and fear of the Lord. Romans 6:2 What shall we then say? Shall we continue to sin, that grace may be abound. Romans 1:32 Who knowing the judgment of God are worthy of death, not only do the same but have pleasure in them that do them.

Where does ones favor go! Has one actually had favor. Where's God? 1 Corinthians 1:20 Where's the wise, where is the disputer of this world? Revelation 17:1 I will show you judgment against the great whore that sitteth upon many great waters. 7:5 For when were in the flesh, {the motions of sins} which were by the law, did the work of our members to bring forth the fruit of death. Motion means a meaningful or expressive change in the position of the body; A gesture. These verses mean. This is done by controlling the captivity of the laws of the mind as written in Romans 7:23 But I see another law in my members, warring against the law of my mind, and bring me into captivity to the law of sin which is my members.

What I am saying, is that one's motions become clogged by being in constant lustful situations of human desire. Which is the law of flesh and death. In psychiatry this is delusional with extreme episodes thereof; The psychotic grandeur of bipolar – schizophrenic deals with the spiritual aspects of ones inability to receive healing. /this is thru the killing of the motions of the Tree of Life meditation systems and any other form of the occult. All are misguided forms of idolatry and perverse forms of spiritualisms as written in Deuteronomy 18:11.

The definition of the word mind is as following as it relates to the law of the mind as it relates to Apostle Paul; {the human consciousness that ignites in the brain and is manifested especially in thought, perception, emotion, will, memory and imagination}.

We fall from grace by connecting motions of sin with others who knowingly assume that they have favor from God. This is basis psychology with lust intentions of the laws of the whore. Romans 1:21 Because when they knew God, they did not retain God in They glorified him not as God, neither were they thankful, but became vain in their imaginations, and their foolish hearts were darkened.

Their Vain is a fruitless outcome with a conceited outlook and approach to God. The tavern whore can be a man or a woman. When you think that you a communicating with a woman, you could be talking to a man. When you think you talking to a man, you are talking to a woman. The Imaginations run wild as they are homosexuals with motions of sin as there representations of lustful burning desires of motions of sin. This includes both male and female prostitute that survey in the temple of God. The church leaders spiritually snare members of the homosexual motion into tempting the entire congregation while inducing their dreams and causing ejaculations in the form of ejaculatory dysfunctions. Perversion is sin. Seduction is sin. Lust is sin and immoral. You see, all of Israel practiced idolatry. There shall be no whoremonger of daughters of the house of Israel nor shall there be a sodomite of the sons of Israel. Exodus 20:5 Thou shall not bow down thyself to worship them nor serve them. By serving their gods man has become motionless

Individuals are vagabonds. They roam from desire to pleasure of the imagination and motion of lust in taverns, pubs and inns. They are sons and daughters of the Devil. Satan is the father of lies as from the beginning he deceived those in the garden as well Cain and Abel. Satan has resurrected himself into modernity by killing God's seed with deception. Revelation 2:24 and have not known the depths of Satan. Yet they are worshippers of Him. Revelations 13:7 The beast was given unto him to make war with the saints of God, and to overcome them: and power was given to him over all kindreds, and tongues, and nations.

This leads to DADT Don't ask don't tell of the uniform code of Military Justice. President Harry S. Truman signed the uniform code of military justice which sets up discharge for homosexual service members. However don't ask don't tell was ignited on December 21, 1993 – September 20, 2011. In 1993 President William J. Clinton endorsed the Bill regarding DADT. You see, 2 Corinthians 10:3-4 For though we walk in the flesh, we do not war after the flesh; [For our weapons of warfare are not carnal, but mighty through God to the pulling down of strongholds. Casting down imaginations of the motions of sin and revenging against sin.

In war, there are motions of sin. The saints of God choose electors by nominating political leaders to rule over nations. For example, leaders of Syria, Afghanistan, Pakistan, Egypt, and Iran are leaders of idolatrous nations. This is not my flesh speaking. This is all theology.

Idolatry has been going on since the beginning of creation. And it has gotten worse. Political leaders have been caught watching pornography and running brothels. For this cause. In John 8:44 Ye are of the father the devil. And the lust of your will do. He was a murderer from the beginning, and abode not the truth, because there is no truth in him. When he speaketh a lie, he speaketh of his own, for he is a liar, and the father of it.

As non devoted to man shall be redeemed. The motions of sin occurs daily but is developed through the seasons as individuals worship times and cycles. All are which are days hours and months by recording their sins on tablets, stone and paper.

In many cases these individuals have an occultic circle of friends. The will of God is grace. Grace has fallen as has the fallen of man. Grace is the Will of God. However, the abusers of the will of God are in totally denial of the resurrection and death of the Lord and Savior.

Meditation and dreams are often used by the addicted. The drug addicted. They have imaginations of the unfruitful. Their desires are very lustful and delusional. Man is in the image of God. In his likeness. However, you cannot fashion an idol to represent any figure, whether it is the form of a, woman, beast and or creature. Anything that is Worshipped other the God is idolatry. Many worship their possessions such as automobiles, money and houses. This is disease oriented and fully brain damaging to the fullest of its meaning. Money is the root of all evil. Man cannot serve two Gods. However, they worship many deities {oracles}, cards and statues!

In addition, meditation is invoked by spiritualists unto the babes of God. Those who look up the spiritualist, king and or queen mother has yet to realize and recognize that he or she is being used as a beast and or tool in shaping the soul of the occultic body. For example, look at the life of Job. Observe how he was scorned daily by the devil. Yet, used by the will of God. Occult groups are filled with gays and lesbians.

A homosexual is a person who is attracted to individuals of the same sexual gender and orientation. We are in a modern form of Sodom and Gomorrah. The perverse has pleasure of the sex toy and or sex doll. Candle worship is relevant in the charmer's vision to seek and call up the dead and or call up ones inner self. In actuality, this is all the aspects of the gay doctrine.

The gay doctrine is filled with one wearing a great amount of jewelry, perfumes and the gay bible. Leviticus 18:22 Man shall not lie with mankind as with a woman, it is an abomination. Neither shall you lie with a beast it is animism. These are works of the people of Canaan and thousands of generations of the Egyptians and Arabs. However, in many Arab nations today individuals are murdered for committing such acts. Iran has more sex changes than any other nation in the world.

A Mukhannathun is one {"male"} who carries his movements in his appearance and in his language as a woman. {INNATE} – not put on by himself. The second type, acts like a woman out of immoral purposes and he is the sinner and blame worthy. Vagabonds are generally of the homosexual drifter they also roam from one crack house to another.

They will turn a trick perversely just for one hit. They are of Satan. John 10:10 The thief, Satan comes to kill steal and destroy anything that has life.

A stronghold is a place of refuge. A stronghold is a location of spiritual wickedness in high places. For example, Something occupied by a special group. For example, seven demons of Beelzebub possessed a man and a child in Matthew and Mark. Beelzebub was known as the prince of demons. In addition, in the demonic realm strongholds exist. The homosexual and perverse form of the demonic occurs whenever individual invoke spirits and omens. Omens are of the devil. Omens cause psychological illnesses and they also cause individuals to imagine the wicked. These are areas in one's life that is occupied and or dominated by a particular group of sin

Church and prostitution has never had grace. The whoremonger is a lustful sinner of the lesbian breed. The motions of sin is high and overly impulsive while it eats the human flesh of others. Circumcision means nothing to God. Deuteronomy 10:16 Circumcise the foreskin your hearts, be no more stiffnecked.

Galatians 6:12 As many as desire to make a fair shew of the flesh, they constrain yo9u to be circumcised; only lest they should suffer persecution for the cross of Christ. Therefore, prostitution is the selling of one's body for money and or drugs. Prostitution is a sin and it is also for the love of sexual pleasure. Prostitution is also a disorder of bipolar.

A whoremonger will seduce you and put a stronghold of weakness upon you. This weakness will cause one to give in unto the seduction of lustful favor. The victim will show favor by giving gifts showing signs of arrogance due to its want of affection. That is willful-sin. The willful-sinner has no mercy. Romans 6: 1-2 Mercy is the Will of God. Do we continue to sin that grace may abound. Prostitution and homosexuality are vile acts of delusional grandeur. The two are connected by extreme means of perverse behaviors and emotions of stronghold. Whenever the two have encounters the orgy of drug addiction manifests itself amongst the entire community.

Spiritual warfare is against any kind of stronghold. Individuals are tamed by the sting of death syndrome. 1 Corinthians 15:55-56 O' death where is thy sting? O' grave where is thy victory? The sting of death is sin. That drug is the injection of death and lust thereof is its' fulfillment of sensual pursuit.

You see, prostitution has corrupted the world since the beginning of creation. Genesis 6:12 And God looked upon the earth, and behold, it was corrupt; for all of the flesh had corrupted his way upon the earth. This world is filled with corrupt leaders of all kind. From clergy to politician all have sinned and com short of the glory of God. Both man and woman are whores of Satan. These things were written in my previous books.

The Devil has been lurking unto the soul and heart of mankind to trigger the syndrome of the spiritual sting of death and will continue reach the soul of the children throughout the world. With deception and lies is how the devil operates. With Ponzi schemes is the devil imposing his will upon its victims. His victims are the saints of God. You see, we can overcome wickedness with prayer and supplication.

Obedience is better than fasting. It is the devil that wants you to be circumcised in order for him to glory off of your flesh. Flesh killeth the spirit and the spirit killeth the flesh of lust thereof. Lust is idolatry and idolatry is sin.

Therefore, sin has got to escape the mindset of the believer. The believer must therefore stand firm against the fruits of the will of the devil. The motion of sin is a divine undertaking against the will of God. A grace abound many, many fall victims to patterns of treachery. This is carried out by vain imaginations which are strongholds. Strong holds are vile acts of motions of sin. Sin is caused by deception and envy. Indeed, vile imaginations of lewdness often leads to sodomy and blasphemy. Corrupt leaders might intrude in my writing in order of keeping their lustful ambitions safe within their environment of darkness. This is where they spy out our liberty in God.

FALLEN

The fall of Satan is evident. Satan is a homosexual. A mukhanathan that takes pride in being gay.

Satan is the father of lies. Harry Truman signed into law a policy that discharged the homosexual from the military. This has lead to the" Don't Ask Don't Tell". Don't' ask don't tell was a bill mandated by former president Bill Clinton to deceive the people into assuming that the laws of God would be pleased with his motives. His motives were to overlook war against Alqaeda and allow Osama Bin Laden to hide throughout the Middle East. This policy was to allows gays in the military.

Isaiah 14:3-5 and 12-15 corrupt individuals fall like Lucifer because of the stronghold of sin. Genesis 4:7Sin is lurking at your door of the believer. Everyone is a Ponzi. What I mean is that everyone is looking for something in a simplistic fashion. Idolatry is a form of simplicity. It is used in schemes of depriving the weak minded. This is by stealing the trust of individuals and gaining their possessions as well as their souls. It is lust of the flesh that causes individuals to have sin in their lives. In sin, many commit adultery, murder and fornication. This includes stealing, corruption and malice.

These are diseases of the soul which enters ones flesh. The fall of Adam occurred because of Eve's deception in the Garden of Eden. Delilah deceived Sampson in the days of the Old Testament. Not to mention the sin of Sodom and Gomorrah. Jeremiah 5:25 your iniquities have turned away these things, and your sins have withheld good things from you. Good things are withheld due to the willful ways of ignorance. This is also done by one deceiving his or her own self by overindulging in unfaithful acts against God.

All things that are done by mankind are not uncovered. Therefore, man has used the way-maker system of tehuti-maat. This is idol worshipping at its utmost. Isaiah 52:9 your iniquities have separated you from your god, your sins have hidden his face from you due to prostitution, homosexuality, drug and sexual abuse. You see, strongholds are difficult to overcome. Ephesians 6:12 For we wrestle not against flesh and blood but against principalities and powers but against rulers of darkness of spiritual wickedness in high places.

You see Satan works in mysterious ways as does God. It was Lucifer who said that he would build his kingdom like God in the book of Daniel and Isaiah. Satan was given authority in revelations, aka the "Mark of the Beast". He was given authority to rule for a certain amount of time and became an arrogant deceiver. All hidden things will be revealed. There is nothing new under the sun. All things that aren't revealed will come to light.

Jeremiah 49:10 but I have made Esau bare, I have his secret places: and he shall not be able to hide himself; his seed is spoiled and his brethren and his neighbors

Occultic members are like Esau. Within Radical Islam, Radical Christianity and the Paut Neteru individuals often change their names and assume other identities to deceive people. They change their names daily, illegally in order to attain success. They assume the identity of others. They change their names monthly by chanting and using omens. They have nicknames which are of the homosexual nature. 2 Corinthians 10:3-4 For though we walk in the flesh, we do not war after the flesh, For our weapons of warfare are not carnal but mighty through the pulling down of strongholds.

Note, I am not denouncing the Ausar Auset Society, Ancient Kemet and or Canaan. As written, the Holy Bible and many other religious groups and organization denounces Egypt, Canaan and ancient Kemet by saying that they were idolatrous and sinful in nature. In restoration, there must be form of equality and a form of non seperative knowledge and understanding of restructuring of the ancient habitats of Ancient Africa / Canaan. Whereas; this world is induced with drug and alcohol addiction. This includes pornography and sex-slave-trade in the areas of academia as well theology, medicine and psychiatry.

Therefore, The Book of Mormon is another theological thought to be criticized. In this, it claims that Joseph Smith is their Holy Prophet. Yet, it has received its prophecy too from ancient Khamit / Canaan. Yes, within its quad, it has books thats have been derived from khamitic names and the consulting of the Metu Neter Oracle - / Umman Thummin that is documented on Exodus.

Lying religions are too substanced induced dogmas that tend to enslave the minds of the weak and lowly by the seeking of tithes and offerings. They say that it is necessary to fast. However, Zacharia 7 / Isaiah 58 mentions that individuals (priests) forced their followers to fast for ungodly purposes. In this, mental illnes has become an epidemic and those who are in a much greater standard of living are guilty of neglectfulness unto to the terminal and mentally disabled.

You see, there are hundreds of personified forms of mental illness. Therefore, there has to be some sort of resurrection of the soul, mind and spirit by rediscovering the self-hidden truths of self-knowledge. Self-knowledge is understanding you ancestry and present. In mental health they diagnose with episodes of delusion and self-pity. However, there are decisions and circumstances that must be tackled daily. In this, there are complications that are coupled with various kinds of mental anguish and pain.

Therefore, with spiritual developing through meditation, these things can be restored with proper nourishment, guidance and understanding. Indeed, racism will never end. It has and was created through slave trade, poverty and urban development. This is modern colonialism. this is more worser than Aparthied. This is corporate and legal genocide. Therefore, have you fallen from grace? Have you ever been given grace. The Bible doesn't tell the entire story correctly.

The Bible was written not for the benefit of all people, especially not for the so-called minority. It was written for the wealthy and cunning. In this, people must understand that there are mental disorders due to spiritual and religious rites in this modern world and satanic age of darkness of which we live.

You see, the Bible and Book of Mormon are books that are illustrious in their {book of fables}! This is the truth. However, I understand that individuals have the right to choose their own path in life. Yet, self-judgement is vital. Individuals become depressed and never know the cause. They have no understanding of the things that are triggering the depressive and manic episodes. Some say that the devil has caused them to do that are inappropriate to the daily standards of the norm. Yet, the norm is not always appropriate for the mental state as well as the spirit and soul.

Individuals fall and fail due to their own conditions and attiudes of self-hatred, depression, hidden angers of aggressions and anxieties. In this, individuals are often secluded to the point of self-expression. Self-expression has been limited to the point of western education. In western education, the talk is non-self-fullfilling. It is generalized through illusions of academia in ways that aren't holistic in nature. This is attained through the animal spirit. within the animal spirit, thoughts are of fancifulness with various forms of of lust and desire.

Lust and desire leads to confusion as written in the Deuteronomy 28:28. This is of the Mosiac Law. This has been stolen by the Hebrew Israelites from the Canaanites and the inhabitants of ancient Khamit.

Genesis 49:26 and Deuteronomy 33:15 / - This has been from the ancient mountians which was taken by the slaver.

You see, confusion causes individuals to become vulnerable when it comes to decision making situations. They are easily swayed into doing ungodly acts. These acts are idolatrous. Idolatrous acts such as; homosexuality, lying, murdering, stealing, cheating and deliberate scapgoating.

Confusion is of various mental disorders. It causes individuals to become diagnosed with major depression disorder as well as bipolar / manic disorder. In this, individuals, certain individuals have with their care pets. Such as birds, cats and or dogs. In addition to this, they aquire various animal diseases. For example, zoonistic disorder and toxoplasmosis are parasitic diseases that generally cause mental illnesses. These mental illnesses are as follows; ADHD, OCD and schizophrenia. These diseases are coupled with individuals having a weakened immune system, inflammation of the brain, affected arteries, HIV, Syphilis and HPV as a result of coming into contact with animal and human feces. In addition, meat eaters can also acquire sexually transmitted diseases and mental illness after eating therof;

Whereas; confusion and mental illness in Deut 28:28 mentions the fact that forms of madness are generalized by disruptions within the neurotransmitters and selective serotonin reuptake inhibitters. Physicians and Psychiatrists say that they are to be stablized with psychotropics and anti-depressants. However, various herbal supplements have been proven to heal the brain receptors as well. DL Phenyalanine and L-Tyrosine as well the herbal form of lithium has been proven to stablize neurotransmitters. In this, libation, meditation, yoga, exercise as well as proper a vegetarian diet will also alter various psychotic episodes of madness, depression, delusion and grandeur.

Sublime thoughts and hallucinations will often occur if there is an extreme form acknowledgement within the realm of receptivity. Receptivity is also known as discernment. In addition, for those reasons, many have been diagnosed with a form or forms of mental disability. The western civilization of the Setien has mentally disabled and caused the blindness to continue for thousands of years up to this current generation of the 21st century. Through deception as false hopes as far as Het Heru Tem Maat is concerned. Therefore vain imaginations occur at a time consuming rate of distraction and distortion of brain cells.

Setiens join aires to seduce unstable individuals with flattery and histrionic delusions that continue to disrupt ones healing process. This is racism. I have seen it as well as been victimized by it.

Whereas; individuals intercede within racial and religious klans to manipulate the lower part of an individuals lower form of intellect. They seduce you when you are vulnurable to manipulation. In this, this has taken prior to the creation of both - the Confederate and America's flag being form. Both of them have mocked and mimmicked God and the African Race. The two are filled and confined with histrionic delusion. In this form of delusion, there are methods of scapegoating and inticement. in inticement there is intimidation and hatred along with segregational forms of grandeur. The mind is highly reprobatable.

Whereas; The slaver provided slaves with military weaponry to create wars so that there were slave wars. Plantation against plantation. This is similar to our current conditions as the government has provided for other nations regarding foreign policies that have enhanced denial, hatred, racism and socialism. This is a continuance from the geneology of the Caucasian, Hebrew, Greek and Arab. In addition, Alexander Stephens of the Whig Party declared that negroes isn't equal to the white man. Slavery is subordination to the superior race is natural to his (the negroe) and normal condition. Also, note; that the negroe has been segregated in the armed forces. As that was once legal within the United States Department of Defence. This also include having been segregated in while incarcerated.

Throughout Vietnam, the hippie movement and civil right movements, there has been a history of drug abuse, sexual addiction and perversions as a result of Jim Crowism and forms of White Supremacy. This includes hatred of the Africans and the African American Race. Whereas; intergration has been a cover-up. Individuals have hidden forms of racism. In their racisms and schemes of life - / they have provided mankind with deception and denial towards social and economical equality by intrusion of our entire being with hypocrisy, arrogance and fraud.

In this, mental illness does have environmental triggers. You are outnumbered amongst certain ethnicities, religious groups and social classes economically. This is when there must be a greater form of understanding of God and the Tree of Life Meditation. In this, there is healing. However, there are scoffers who will by fallacious towards themselves as well as others. Racism is persistant and a condition behavior that is taught and trained by the ancestry of those who had already invaded ancient Egypt (Kemet) and Canaan. For this is in chapters nine and ten in the King James Version of the Holy Bible.

Racism is economical and destroying the impoverished. You see, The Caucasian is of the queer as folk. They have a so-called keen eye of the capacity of seeing the future. They're Setiens and are evil doers by worshipping forms of Gay Tarot and WICCA! This is abominable.

In addition, tarot cards do not allow individuals to work on their individualized destiny through meditation and spiritual work. However, they are fortune telling objects that were created by the Godwin Group which studies the European Tetragrammaton as forms of Judaism. However, it is used by psychics and mediums throughout the world. This particular system does not heal ones destiny, mental, behavioral and or spiritual conditions. It provides information regarding regarding a quick fixed solution that is needed to fulfill fleshy desires of the heart.

This is through the lusts and greed of the Jew, Greek and Caucasian. Also, many people have fallen into this category of darkness of the Gestalt Theory. This theory was created by Laura Perls during her exile from Germany which led her to migrate to Africa to evaluate Africans in order to create a variety of exams for individuals with patterns of learning and mental disability.

Poet and spiritualist, Author Edward Waite created an esoteric and masonic tarot card deck called The Kaballah (Rider-Waite - Tarot Deck). However, it doesn't assist in the healing of behavioral patterns and negative spiritual conditions. It too is a fortune telling device. Unlike the Kemetic Tree of Life, it doesn't deal with dietary, health and spiritual laws. It is another model of the quick fortune telling and quick-hitting (crack deal) and or human form of sin and scandal. This is a scandal of David Godwin. Godwin was the author of the Cabalistic Encylopedia.

You see, the Holy Bible sanctions such use of those objects. However, The European has gotten away with this. Yet, the have denounced the African ways of living by changing the truth into lies with their mockery of God with their idolatrous conditions and behavioral patterns.

In this, The Mental Measurment Yearbook is yet another method of twisting the African, minority and foreigner in The united States of America. The education system has failed to understand the actual spirit, soul, mind and destiny of its deciples / pupils. Therefore, deciples are students. However, Jesus had twelve deciples were Caucasian and he was a so-called Jew. Did his messengers deceive the people, the world and the societies of which they had lived. Indeed they did. Their messages were inconsistent and fallacious.

Therefore, read with an understanding. Whereas, The Holy Bible is based on Judaism, Christianty and Islam of the Western Civilization. They were all derived form Kemet and Canaan. In ancient times Canaan was Palestine west of the Jordan River. The nations of Canaan were seven in number. They were;

1. Canaanites
2. Hittites

3. Hivites

4. Perizzites

5. Girgashites

6. Amorites

7. Jubusites

Yet, The Holy Bible Denounces those particular nations in Deuteronomy 20:17 it mentions that those nations shall be utterly destroyed. This is hatred and racism. For those purposes, there is fighting in Africa and the Middle East today. Racism has caused wars, slave wars and wars against the America!

Rascism and hatred and idolatry are causes and forms of mental illness. Genesis 13:7 prior to the fall of Sodom, Gomorrah and other cultures there was no idolatry. A lord is a British Monarch from the UK. This of which is defined as a ruler, king and or judge of a particular nation and or province. For this purpose, racism had to have existed along religious and psychiatrical lines for thousands of years after the invasion and conquering of ancient Kemet and Canaan as well as the slaves throughout Africa!

Mental illness and racism are coupled by them hating you as they follow your every step in life. This is mere and moreso hypocrisy. Racism, mental illness and hatred are also written in Deuteronomy 7:1 of Judaism which is geered towards the Ancient Egyptian (Khamit / Canaan. Racism is not necessary hatred. It is based on fear. The enemy and racism are coupled with lies and deception. In this, there is a sense of delusion, histrionic and granduer. This means that the caucasian has been in denial for millions of years due to their false notions of white supremacy. In white supremacy there is the attitude that the white man is greater than any other race of people. Ezra 9:1-2 mentions the intermingled African nations have been seduced by self-indulging pleasures of idolatry as it relates to paganism and polytheistic religious beliefs and behavorial patterns.

Therefore, the exceptional person has been denied access towards all forms of equality. In social equality there is love, patience and understandings that everyone is equal. Who are you fooling? This is a fantasy. There has been many psychological examinations that have deludged the history of great African nations and its heritage. For this, we have been pleasured with deceit and hatred. We've been deceived by words of seduction and pleasures of the goddamn setien.

A system that has been designed to de-empower the dispersed African nations due the so-called sins of Adam and Eve. You see, those two weren't the first human beings on the civilization. Zinjanthropus verses the white man and his racist rants that has been a cancer to the human mind, spirit and soul since the conception of the universe. Meaning, we as a people must recognize that facts that homosexualism and racism are immortal plagues that millions of people have brought against and amongst themselves. Whereas; there are professionals who are to assist others in facilitating their lives. However, they have fallen into the shadows of desperate and racy schemes of pleasure with their cunning and sensual perversions of dogma by comforting their selfish forms of lustful deeds of vile affection with unnatural affections.

This is just stubborness as well as selfishness as the negroe has been deceived, manipulated and denied as God by the Shemites, Japhites and their current children of this generation. Lies can be immortal. Education can be immortal. Wisdom can be immortal as well as lies, hypocrisy, racism, substance abuse, GLBT and hatred.

This is my question as the Greeks and Judaism had written the Holy Bible. Whereas, Alexander The Great was bisexual as well as individuals in the Confederacy, Civil War and Union Armies were living idolatrous lives under the table. Was this known as the "Fraudulent Enlistment" and later considered DADT. Individials who were gay and or bisexual were paired in military bunks as this was considered a "Jewel" - by mating and pairing the gays this would create a strong sense of joy amongst the troops as they were pleased by the norm of this vile form of wickedness.

DEALING WITH THE REALITY OF YOUR BEHAVIOR

The power of white racism economically through health care and livinging conditions has strictly enslaved the entire nature of the neurological system. In this, Kenya awards same-sex relationships with harsh methods of capital punishment / meaning torture. In the majority of the African continent, acts of LGBTQ are sanctioned. Therefore, the individual must deal with the realities of his or her sinful behaviors and idolatrous activities.

Racism and homosexuality has hit the spine, spirit and soul of the African Ancestry. In addition, the negroe has been tormented by the wickedness of the European ancestory. First they were pagan, GLBT as well as cannibals as to beastializing animals with perversive sexual activities and whoredoms. This is a shameful pollution, genocide of humanity. You see, we are a blind race, religion and culture. Homosexuality is a neurotic behavior that man can and will not repair due to its arrogance and disregard towards its own lies regarding the humanial affairs. Homosexuality is a behavior that can be innate or learned.

In this, behavior is a combined verb/noun. Therefore, the be in behavior means to be as to an occurance and the havior is coined as the action or situation that can be either exist as a result of internalized or externalized life-forces that are manifested within the individuals mind and or physical existing surroundings. Therefore, as we live in a physical or metaphysical realm of life, we are sometimes influenced by the endocrine system as well as the entire nervous system. This is where psychiatry and metaphysical sciences are formed. You see, our mind and spirits are governed by the conscious and subconscious realms. Note: see psychiatry and the Tree of Life Meditation System all volumes by Ra n Nefer Amen I.

In addition, for nearly a century, the Buros Institute has creation the Mental Measurement Yearbook series of psychological assessment that is based on creating test manuals for assessing individuals with special needs. This too is culturally bias as the testing tools aren't properly provided for all cultures. They assess indiviuals based on their knowledge of testing and not on their knowledge lacking therof with regards to each individuals divine destiny -/ purpose as spiritual developmental make-up as the Afrocentric spiritual systems have.

These forms of testing only enhance the vulnarability of individuals - towards lacking self-esteem and the motivation crime, poverty, perversions and homosexuality. Within the BDIS The Behavior Disorders Identification Scales there is no justification that this will enable the impoverish to overcome. As a result of poverty, this doesn't actually mean that they are lacking knowledge of holistic behavioral methods that are intended. It is a known fact that the test have been created by scholarly Europeans in the field of Egyptology, Greek mythology, psychometry, psychiatry and education.

You see, those individuals are wealthy and have been awarded with monetary relics to enable them to research specific cultures, religions and races. Specifically, the African and Dominican Republica. This is the ways in which theorist theorize and evaluate individuals for their unethical findings. Therefore, this is why slavery was intended. Within slavery, there are several acts of pervasives. Which includes mental bondage as a result of operant conditioning.

Therefore; this has lead to self-centered risks that are and were taking by the slaver who molested the child, raped the mother and or father and canabbilzed / maimed many by torture. Mental as well as physical torture had taken place and is currently shaping the progress of the world. Individuals were starved and often ate each. They often urinated as well manured on each other while suffering unhumane treament on slaveships by the slaver. This is known as ENURESIS.

See; the Gaulites, Greeks and Romans. This is written in throughout the book of Numbers, Leviticus and Deuteronomy as well as the first six chapters of Romans in the King James Version of The Bible. You see, behaviors are taught, trained and instilled within the conscious and subconscious of individuals. Behaviors are then imitated by triggered by many. These then become diagnoses of a variety of mental and or medical illnesses that are often both untamable and uncurable.

GLBTQ, for example, are coordinated by actions and inactions of the reptillian and mammallian parts of the brain. Therefore, the GLBTQ gay, lesbian, bisexual, transgendered and queer have been imitating and loquacious individuals throughout their lives. As they are currently teaching Queer Education to children in classrooms and churches throughout The United States of America. The Caucasian is the creator of Gay activisim.

Perversion is an appetite for lustfulness. Such as drugs and other illegal substances. This is mindboggling to the root of the worlds history. Orgys by the Greeks and Romans during Christendom and the conquering of ancient Egypt and Canaan by the Philistine, Jew and Arab. Therefore, neurosis in homosexuality often leads to children born with many kinds of deformity.

Hosea (:16-17) I will slay their cherished offspring. My God will reject them because they have not obeyed him; they will be wanderers among nations. As mentioned in Numbers 23:9 I see a people who do not even know themselves. This leads to the fact of cerebral vascular disease due to cocaine induced hypertension that leads to low birth wieght due to maternal smoking. In addition, any form of oxy - also causes depressions and various forms of anxiety due to neurological dysfunctions and brain diseases along the line of the following; ANS, CNS and PNS.

In many cases, these are self induced neurological disease that are caused by carelessness of the birthing parents. There are several diseases that are triggered / passed on to the offspring as a result of addictions to drugs and prescribed medications. You see, Deut

28:59 mentions that there will be lingering illnesses and plagues that will be extremly severe. Whereas; in most cases, individuals suffer from forms of Neuropsychiatric Monism as they are diseases of the nervous system that often cause manic depressive diseases that are neurological and neuromuscular diseases.

These neurological diseases are caused by syphilis of the spine and diabetic ovarian. In this, this eventually causes Parkinson's Disease due to syphilis dementia and early onsets of dementia. Congenital Syphilis by the uterus and utero are stages of cancer.

Due to diabetic mitochondrial diseases individuals have hereditary metabolic diseases that are in the family of anemia / anemic - sickel cell, TB which eventually leads to blindness. There are also stages of alcoholic psychosis with the development of genetic seizures. In this, individuals have galactosemia where they need milk and dairy substitutes that will assist them in calcuim and protein intake.

As previously mentioned, infants and infants and adults have congestive heart failure due to drug addiction. This is Inherited Hyperammonemias. This is also when diabetic neuropathies occur as blood sugra levels are inconsistent when taking nitro glycerine. Therefore, children are inherited with epilepsy, drug resistent seizures as infants are born prematurly.

In addition, pituitary gland disorders lead to aggression in childhood diabetes due to high blood pressure and lactational urine contractions. Children later develope ADHD as physicians have to have knowledge of the failing psychological and IQ tests. Otherwise, this can lead to various forms of dsylexia, auditory and or visual lacks. Individuals are very seldom diagnosed with Gerstmann Syndrome. This is where writing, mathematics, reading left - to - right and recognition are difficult. This is neurological.

In some cases, psychiatric assistance is required and yet helpful. However, one must recognized his or her own needs. Nefer Amen, "they manipulate the lower part of you being". Therefore, the activity of the schizophrenic is limited by humanity. This is handicap discrimination. Psychiatry has claimed that DD Delusional Disorder is of others. Such as Bipolar, Schizophrenic and or Hebephrenic (Paranoia).

Poorly being diagnosed individuals are later coined with the diagnosis of PPD Purified Protein Disorders leading to and later as a result of bizarre behaviors, inappropriate emotions, anxiety vs. panic attacks of psycho-neurosis and thyroid psychosis. All mental illnesses are neurological. Adjustment disorders as well as cognitive disorders are from anxieties of zenophobia.

The reality of zenophobia is the fact that individuals have fears of a particular sexual gender, religion, race and of the unknown. In this, individuals slander whatever they cannot comprehend as well as others through jealousy, hatred and racial discrimination. Therefore, they tend to have neurological disorders of the frontal lobe. In this disorder, there are forms of lobotomy (pituitary disorders) that eventually leads to insomnia, forms of manic depressive diseases and hyperactivity syndrome due to frontal lobe lesions.

One must also note the fact that individuals become loquatious with a confused mental state as well as having the inconsistency within the thought and mind. Confusion is often triggered by prefrontal parts of the frontal lobe. This is when individuals tend to prophecy which is in regards to his or her past, present and future events the are within the modernity of ones' life. Meaning, thoughts often become patterns of religious and or spiritual that is within IV DSM revised edition - / page 685 - V62.89.

Religious and or spiritual concepts and or connections that are leading and relating to false and hypocritical themes of fanciful, delusional and granduer. This is consistent with fanciful hopes of a false and delusional saviour and being saved by a western form of thought and religion. Therefore, in psychiatry, there are themes and concepts in which individuals are often diagnosed by psychiatrist who have what is known as the zenophobic effect. In this, the African and African American has been observed for thousands of years and evaulated negatively by Egyptologist / Greeks, Arabs, Christian and the Jew.

This is a psychological betrayal of the entire neurological development of the African - Black scholar and human. This too has become economical due to the disinfranchisment of the poor by mercenaries who had taught us how to pray and yet to conquer and divide us - / then take our entire culture and heritage. Therefore, this has lead to deceitfulness amongst the highly regarded and so-called educated and intellectual bigots. Of the inclusion of the cunning schemer of the perpretration of the fraud, idolatry, beastiality, incest, GLBTQ and political scam through a ponzy.

We have been enslaved by ponzy organizers and zonophobics until we have and formed a genocidal affect on our own people. We are a blind people. We are seeking things through works of the setien. This is a term that is coined as the Devil. Therefore, Judiasm, LDS, Jehovha's Witness, Christianity and Islam have consulted and joined aires to abolish African spirituality by seducing the minds of those who will change them indirectly as long as there is something lustful and deceitful within it for them.

We are a pleasure seeking people who are lost and fooled by ourselves. We are to blame only ourselves for our lack of growth and stability within the brain, spirit and soul. The Asian, Arab and Whity are as well, too guilty. As negative behaviours have manifested and have been well documented as psychiatric disorders by the GLBTQ and white-man every since we met in the beginning.

Whereas; zenophobic behavior is a form of racism throughout the methods of racial profiling of which is a form of heredity. Whereas Exodus chapter 3 explains the concept of Moses being annointed by a Hebraic God to kill, steal and destroy the people of Canaan as well as his fellow Egyptian in order to gain prosperity within the lines of Canaan and Etc. All of which coincides with my notion of the Caucasian, Asian, Arab and Greek commiting an organized form of genocide against the People of Alkabulan / Kemet and Canaan.

This is a major genocide, hatred and bigotry against our present and future generations of the liberation of the African people at the hands of the slaver. This is as a result of the conception of genetic and heredity at the hands of the delusional and wicked ancestry of racial lines of the greedy and barbaric devils / setiens from the European nations as well as the Asiatic and Arabs conquestidors of the Middle and Atlantic Passages of prowess.

In this, the behavior of PPD has been devloped as a result of shame and doubt with regards to one's particular race as forms of physhological testing had been practiced to create, induce and monitor a so-called nigga into becoming a bonified - certified fool. As be-havior is a verb as well as a noun and a plural. This is created. Has been created to inform mankind that actions taken can be internal as well as external. Therefore these are mechanisms with the brain in its entirity. As behaviors can be innate and slave-like and or taught or learned.

Whereas; teaching is to train as animals through mental bigotry and within the lines of cleverness of the intelligent setien. This is which is the Westernized political and educational establishment of the Parlimentry / European concepts of masonic rule of within the royal line the Scots and those of Great Britian. They considered us as heathens and pagans. You see, they enslaved us and created monoplies of mental and spiritual control as methods of sociology and philosophical methods of manipulating individuals with various forms of tools of shaping and manipulating our behaviours within the creation of psychiatry.

The human behavior has been believed to be influenced by the endocrine and nervous systems. However, I beg to differ with those concepts of science. In this, within neurology (BRAIN) is the only and key ingredient to the possible solution of healing and curing the nicotine and drug infested - alcoholic induced psychotic. Read for yourselves. Find your niche. You'll see that you hold the key to your own successes and failures in your walk towards divinity.

Therefore; racism is a mental defect that recognizes the truth, right and wrong. However, transforms all into lies as the devil / setein did when he devoured Ausar into fourteen pieces. You see, the Bible and Quran were written with slavery on the minds of their writers. They created ways of enslavement. Not only in a physical sense. In a mental state as well as them creation of laws towards the establishment of their control. That is the European and Arab / Jew.

This goes for lack of employment to lower wages for the so-called economically disadvantaged races. This includes all Africans and African Americans. Africans were in America beyond 25 B.C.E. Homesexuality was never practiced amongst the African until they were introduced during slavery by the European.

There is another form of psychosis. Which is called Phantosmia. Phantosmia is a variety of perverse hallucinations due to the lack of understanding and misconception of all of the spheres on the Khamitic Tree of Life initiation and meditation system. Note: one must acquire this gift in order to in order to maintain steadfast within all undertakings and processes that life brings upon him or her. This includes racism.

Therefore, you cannot like one diety and dislike another. You cannot be prejudice towards one diety and affirmate another. That is The Khaibit level of the western cultures of the Arab, Jew and Christian. They are segregative in their thought process as is the Caucasian and many uncle Tom's and house-Nigs are.

Printed in the United States
By Bookmasters